FIRST PLACE™

LEADER'S GUIDE

A CHRIST-CENTERED HEALTH PROGRAM

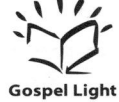
Gospel Light

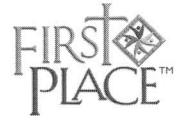
FIRST PLACE™

Gospel Light is an evangelical Christian publisher dedicated to serving the local church. We believe God's vision for Gospel Light is to provide church leaders with biblical, user-friendly materials that will help them evangelize, disciple and minister to children, youth and families.

It is our prayer that this Gospel Light resource will help you discover biblical truth for your own life and help you minister to others. May God richly bless you.

For a free catalog of resources from Gospel Light, please contact your Christian supplier or contact us at 1-800-4-GOSPEL or www.gospellight.com.

PUBLISHING STAFF
William T. Greig, Publisher
Dr. Elmer L. Towns, Senior Consulting Publisher
Pam Weston, Senior Editor
Patti Pennington Virtue, Associate Editor
Jeff Kempton, Editorial Assistant
Hilary Young, Editorial Assistant
Kyle Duncan, Associate Publisher
Bayard Taylor, M.Div., Senior Editor, Biblical and Theological Issues
Dr. Gary S. Greig, Senior Advisor, Biblical and Theological Issues
Barbara LeVan Fisher, Cover Designer
Samantha A. Hsu, Designer

ISBN 0-8307-2867-8
© 2001 First Place
All rights reserved.
Printed in the U.S.A.

All Scripture quotations, unless otherwise indicated, are taken from the *Holy Bible, New International Version*®. Copyright © 1973, 1978, 1984 by International Bible Society. Used by permission of Zondervan Publishing House. All rights reserved.

Other version used is:

KJV—King James Version. Authorized King James Version.

CAUTION

The information contained in this book is intended to be solely informational and educational. It is assumed that the First Place participant will consult a medical or health professional before beginning this or any other weight-loss or physical fitness program.

COPYRIGHT NOTICE

ABOUT THE AUTHORS

As the National Director of First Place, **Carole Lewis** is a renowned conference speaker, author and retreat leader specializing in the area of fitness and nutrition. She is the author of *Choosing to Change* and *First Place.* She has been the full-time director of the program since 1987.

Kay Smith is the Associate National Director of First Place. She has been a full-time staff member of Houston's First Baptist Church since 1988. In addition to speaking at retreats, seminars and conferences, Kay writes a monthly article for the First Place newsletter.

Nancy Taylor has been the National Leadership Training Director for First Place since 1997. She teaches leadership principles to First Place leaders throughout the country, writes a monthly newsletter article and speaks at First Place workshops, rallies and conferences.

CONTENTS

WELCOME TO FIRST PLACE

WHAT IS FIRST PLACE?

The First Place program is the result of a godly desire placed in the hearts of a group of Christians. This desire was to establish a Christ-centered weight-control program. The basic question that initiated the search for such a program was, "Since God has saved us from our sins and given us abundant life, why can't we, as Christians, use that same power in the area of weight control?"

With that question in mind, they decided to develop a program that would meet the needs of Christians in the area of weight control. Little did they know what they were undertaking! It was an immense assignment, but knowing God had called them to the task, they placed all of their hopes and aspirations in Him and began the project. They prayed, studied, prayed, read, prayed and wrote, and First Place began to take shape!

They knew that in order to be effective, the program had to focus totally on the Lord and include Bible study, small-group support and accountability, a proven common-sense nutrition plan, exercise, a method of record keeping and many other elements. They knew putting Christ first in their lives would be the success of the program. Their aim was for growth in all areas: spiritual, mental, emotional and physical.

Matthew 6:33, "Seek ye first the kingdom of God, and his righteousness; and all these things shall be added unto you" (*KJV*), was chosen as the theme verse for the program. Hence, the name "First Place."

The original First Place groups met in March of 1981 at First Baptist Church of Houston, Texas. What began as a Christ-centered weight-loss program has evolved into a nationally recognized total health program. Today, the First Place program is used in every state and many foreign countries. Thousands of lives have been radically changed by the power of Christ.

We praise God for the leadership He provided as all steps of First Place were planned and penned. Our greatest desire was, and continues to be, that God will receive all the glory, honor and praise, and that as a result of First Place, individuals will live healthier, happier and more abundant lives with God as their first priority.

The goal of First Place is for balance in the spiritual, mental, emotional and physical areas of a person's life. Meeting weekly in groups of up to 20 people, First Place members stay with the same group for the entire 13 weeks. Each meeting includes nutritional information, class discussion, Bible study and prayer. The Live-It plan is based on the USDA Food Guide Pyramid. Using behavior modification techniques and the Nine Commitments, members learn how to be victorious over past eating patterns and to commit their minds—and ultimately their bodies—to God.

Upon entering the program, members agree to the following Nine Commitments:

1. **ATTEND** a meeting each week.
2. **ENCOURAGE** one person in your class weekly.
3. **PRAY** daily.
4. Commit to daily **BIBLE READING**.
5. **MEMORIZE** one Scripture passage weekly.
6. Complete a weekly **BIBLE STUDY**.
7. Follow the First Place **LIVE-IT PLAN**.
8. Keep a First Place **COMMITMENT RECORD**.
9. **EXERCISE** three to five times weekly.

WHY CHOOSE FIRST PLACE?

Health Benefits
- Weight loss, resulting from a balanced plan consisting of healthy food and exercise
- A proven health plan that benefits those with health concerns such as hypertension, heart disease, cancer, diabetes and lower back pain

Discipleship
- Balanced lifestyle through Bible study, prayer, Scripture reading and memorization
- Accountability through small-group support

Outreach
- Attracts the unchurched
- Provides many opportunities to share Christ

WHO JOINS FIRST PLACE?

Those Desiring to Lose Weight Who
- Struggle with losing 5 to 10 pounds
- Battle obesity
- Are tired of yo-yo dieting

Those Desiring to Achieve a Healthier Lifestyle Through
- Gaining knowledge in nutrition
- Implementing a consistent exercise plan
- Developing a healthy lifestyle for their entire family

Those Desiring to Be a Part of a Support Group Who
- Need accountability
- Seek support through prayer
- Experience similar struggles

WHEN DOES FIRST PLACE MEET?

A Year-Round Program Consisting Of
- Four 13-week sessions
- Weekly meetings of one hour and 15 minutes

Any Day or Time
- Weekday morning, noon or evening classes
- Saturday classes
- Sunday classes

WHERE DOES FIRST PLACE MEET?

CHURCH CLASSROOM	WORKPLACE	HOME	FITNESS CENTER	CAMPUS

USING THE *FIRST PLACE* LEADER'S GUIDE

HELPING OTHERS GIVE CHRIST FIRST PLACE

As a First Place leader, you have the opportunity to help others put Jesus Christ in first place in their lives. As the Lord works in people's lives, they will grow spiritually and make progress in reaching their weight-loss goals.

The Bible studies your group members complete each week will help them learn more about Christ and what it means for Him to be in first place in their lives. Individual study is only the first step in the learning process. Life change comes as group members meet together; share ideas, insights and struggles; affirm and encourage one another; and support one another in prayer. As a leader, you play a vital role in the learning process. This *First Place Leader's Guide* will help you to lead your group in a positive time of learning that will become a highlight of your weekly time together.

A CAFETERIA LINEUP OF LEARNING ACTIVITIES

The *First Place Leader's Guide* is designed like a cafeteria with lots of choices. But just like a cafeteria, you don't need to choose everything! Each weekly session contains more questions and activities than you will have time to complete. Pick and choose what relates best to your particular group. As you learn more about the individuals in your group, you will be able to tailor your sessions to meet their needs.

BUILDING ON A FOUNDATION OF INDIVIDUAL STUDY

The Bible study that members complete during the week provides the foundation for learning. The *First Place Leader's Guide* assumes group members have completed their personal study and are ready to discuss what they have learned during the weekly group session. Explain to your group about the importance of the group session as a time for further learning as members share the insights and questions that grew out of their personal study. Your group will tend to do what you expect them to do. Set high standards and they will meet them.

A FELLOW STRUGGLER—NOT THE RESIDENT EXPERT

Don't try to be the person with every answer. Don't be afraid to say: "I don't know." "That's a great question." "Can anyone else help us?" Be yourself. Share your life and your struggles. Let your group see the difference Jesus Christ is making in your life as you strive to put Him in first place.

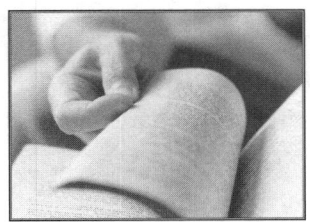

Getting Started

STEP-BY-STEP

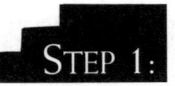 **STEP 1:** LEARN MORE ABOUT FIRST PLACE

Leadership Materials

1. The First Place Group Starter Kit is available to aid in beginning a new group. It includes the following components:

   - *First Place Leader's Guide*
   - *First Place Member's Guide*
   - *Giving Christ First Place* Bible study (including the Scripture Memory CD)
   - *First Place* by Carole Lewis with W. Terry Whalin
   - *Choosing to Change* by Carole Lewis
   - *Nine Commitments* Video
   - *Food Exchange Plan* Video
   - *Orientation* Video

2. If a church wants to offer more than one group at a time, a separate *First Place Leader's Guide* should be purchased for each additional group leader. Additional Group Starter Kits are not necessary. All of the other components are available for individual purchase as well.

Do Leaders Need Training?

1. Training is beneficial but not required.
2. Leadership experience can be gained by participation in a First Place group if one is available in your area.
3. The Group Starter Kit contains the essentials needed to lead a group, including videos to help you understand the program.
4. For information regarding training opportunities, call the First Place national office or access the First Place website.

Where Do I Get Additional Information?

1. First Place national office: 1-800-727-5223
2. First Place website: www.firstplace.org
3. First Place monthly newsletter

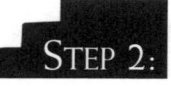 ## STEP 2: REQUEST PERMISSION TO BEGIN

1. Make an appointment with your pastor or other appropriate staff member to share information and present materials for review. Communicate that the First Place program can be
   a. An outreach tool;
   b. A ministry of discipleship;
   c. A health program for all members.
2. Discuss
   a. First Place materials costs (and explain the program is designed to recover any costs incurred by the church);
   b. Possible meeting days and times;
   c. Child care availability and costs.

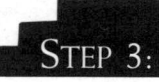 ## STEP 3: RECRUIT AND PREPARE LEADERS

Looking for Leaders

1. A potential leader is one who
   a. Has a desire to minister in the area of total wellness.
   b. Is willing to facilitate a small group.
2. When developing First Place leadership, we suggest
   a. One leader and one assistant for each group of up to 20 people.
   b. Each member should be viewed as a potential future leader.

3. When choosing an assistant or coleader, we suggest
   a. Someone who is able to come early;
   b. Someone who has completed one 13-week session of First Place and shows an interest in continuing;
   c. Someone with leadership potential or abilities;
   d. Someone who is friendly and can easily communicate with others;
   e. Someone who is dependable and discreet.

Optional Leadership Responsibilities

The following duties could be assigned to group members as needed (or used to train or evaluate potential leaders):

1. Weigh members before class starts, allowing the leader freedom to meet and greet members as they arrive.
2. Make name tags.
3. Encourage absentee members through phone calls, e-mails and/or notes.
4. Help evaluate the Commitment Records (CRs).

Training

1. First Place workshops are one-day events with basic training for new leaders and creative teaching ideas for experienced leaders.
2. First Place conferences offer leadership seminars for new and experienced leaders.
3. Fitness Weeks also provide basic training for new leaders.
4. Opportunities for training may be obtained through calling the First Place national office or accessing the First Place website.

Support

1. A church with more than one leader should organize a leaders' group for prayer, support and accountability.
2. Area leaders' meetings are available in some regions. Check the First Place website or newsletter for scheduled meetings.

STEP 4: SCHEDULE DATES AND TIMES FOR YOUR MEETINGS

1. Consider the dates and times convenient for the leader and potential members.
2. Check church calendar for specific dates and available classroom space. Or investigate the use of other facilities, such as workplaces, community centers, etc.
3. Consider need and availability of child care when selecting the day and time of class.

STEP 5: DETERMINE THE COST TO MEMBERS

Consider charging $10 to $20 more than the cost of the materials and using the additional monies collected to cover items such as:

- Shipping fees
- An upright medical scale for weekly weigh-ins
- Child care
- The victory celebration
- Fitness testing
- Additional resources (e.g., books, food models and other instructional items)
- First Place materials for the leader and assistant leader
- Leadership training

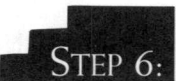

STEP 6: PURCHASE FIRST PLACE MATERIALS

Where
- At your local Christian bookstore
- Through Gospel Light at 1-800-4GOSPEL or www.gospellight.com
- From First Place at www.firstplace.org

When
- Order materials at least two weeks early if you plan to make them available at orientation.

—OR—

- Order materials *after* the orientation meeting—two weeks *prior* to your first meeting. When purchasing from your local bookstore, call ahead with the Bible study selection to insure adequate stock.

What
1. Each group member needs the following:
   a. One Member Kit, which includes the following:
      - *First Place Member's Guide*
      - Four motivational audiocassettes
      - *First Place Journal*
      - *First Place Scripture Memory Verses: Walking in the Word*
      - One 13-pack of Commitment Record cards

   Option: Couples might share one Member Kit.

   b. One Bible study book which includes the following:
      - Ten weeks of daily Bible study
      - Six Wellness Worksheets
      - Scripture memory verse CD bound inside the back cover
      - Prayer Request pages
      - 13 Commitment Records
      - Leader Discussion Guide

2. Each continuing class member only needs one new Bible study book.

BIBLE STUDY SELECTIONS

Giving Christ First Place—Members will learn how to give Christ first place, the importance of prayer, the joy of obeying God, the truth about excuses, how to cope with temptations, the secrets of true satisfaction, pleasing God and committing to do His will.

Everyday Victory for Everyday People—Members learn that many of their compulsions and everyday battles are spiritual warfare and must be fought with the spiritual weapons of daily prayer and Bible study.

Life Under Control—Members learn that with God's supernatural power, they can gain control in every aspect of life: thoughts, emotions, actions, relationships, spoken words and eating habits.

Life That Wins—Members obtain a deeper understanding of God's grace, His unconditional love, His perfect plan and powerful provision. Through the development of the Christlike qualities of the fruit of the Spirit, members learn how to win.

Seeking God's Best—God wants His best for our lives! Often God's best is hidden behind circumstances or relationships that appear good. In choosing the good, we might miss God's best. Members are challenged to ask God to give them a desire for His best.

Pressing On to the Prize—The goal of pressing on toward God's purpose requires a power beyond our human capabilities. This study will help individuals discover God's enabling power in their daily lives.

Pathway to Success—This study challenges members to begin the journey of success through a practical look at the qualities and behaviors that produce growth in the Christian life.

Living the Legacy—You have an inheritance as a child of the King! Your spiritual blessings include being chosen, loved, adopted, predestined and forgiven. This study helps members live a life worthy of their calling as children of God.

Why Publicize?

1. To introduce First Place to
   - Church members
   - Coworkers
   - The whole community
   - The unchurched
2. To preregister alumni members

When to Publicize

Begin publicity one month before orientation.

Where to Publicize

- Church bulletin and/or announcements
- Church newsletter
- Local newspaper
- Radio
- Information table
- Sunday School and/or Bible study small groups
- Posters in businesses and libraries

What to Publicize

- Date, time and location for the orientation meeting
- Date, time and location of classes
- Contact person and phone number

How to Publicize

Describe First Place as a Christ-centered health program with an emphasis on weight control. Inform your church and community that First Place is designed to help people develop balance in their lives: spiritually, emotionally, mentally and physically.

- Submit an article to the church newsletter, Sunday bulletin, community newsletter or local newspaper (see sample, p. 76).
- Advertise on local television and radio stations.
- Mail preregistration letters to alumni (see sample, p. 79).
- Distribute flyers (see samples, pp. 75-77).
- Provide personal testimonies in worship services, Sunday School or local media. Or use the 30- or 60-second promo portion of the *Orientation* video in the Group Starter Kit.
- Display posters in local business establishments or local libraries.
- Set up a display of First Place materials in the church foyer.

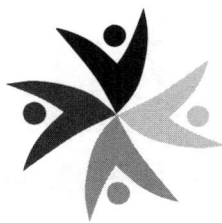

Note: Publicity should clearly inform people that the orientation is essential for new-member registration. An orientation includes a presentation of the First Place program, the Nine Commitments and testimonies. At the orientation meeting, potential members should be shown the *Orientation* video and then given the opportunity to register for the upcoming session.

STEP 8: PREREGISTER ALUMNI

When you plan a new session, contact all former First Place members about your upcoming session. A sample letter is on page 79. Send information well in advance of the orientation. Orientation is not required for alumni, but some may choose to come for motivation and inspiration or to bring a friend. The preregistration form for alumni is found on page 80.

STEP 9: PLAN AND PRESENT ORIENTATION

- Enlist others to help with the orientation.
- Set a date and time. It is best to schedule the orientation two weeks prior to the first class.
- Consider scheduling more than one orientation time.
- Reserve a place for the meeting and secure any necessary equipment (e.g., TV and VCR).
- Set up a table to display First Place materials.
- Make copies of the registration forms (p. 78) for new members.
- Make copies of the Member Survey (p. 88) to give out at registration.
- Show the *Orientation* video.
- Provide registration information.

ORIENTATION AGENDA

I. **Welcome and Opening Prayer**

II. **Testimony**
    Encourage First Place members to give a personal testimony of how First Place has impacted their lives. You may plan one or more testimonies to be given before the video. Testimonies may relate to one or more of the commitments.

III. **Play the *Orientation* Video**
     Cue video to the *Orientation* before meeting begins.

IV. **Registration Information**
    A. Classes Offered
       Announce beginning/ending dates of session and the day and time of each class.
    B. Program Costs
       Explain to the members the cost of the materials they will receive. Give details of child care, if available.

V. **Questions and Answers**
    Allow time at the end of Orientation for questions relating to information presented. If questions become too long or too personal, offer to meet with that person at the end of the meeting.

VI. **Commitment Time**
    A. Prayer
       Lead the group in a prayer, asking God for strength to keep the commitments.
    B. Registration
       Ask them to complete registration forms and sign the commitment. Collect the registration forms and fees.

STEP 10: ORGANIZE CLASSES

If you will have more than one group, divide registration forms into groups according to day and time each member selected. Prepare a roster for each group as illustrated below. Make copies of the roster for each group member. Distribute these at the first group meeting.

<u>Sample</u>

FIRST PLACE ROSTER

Session _January–March, 2001_ Class Day ___Tuesdays___ Class Time ___7:00 p.m.___

Name	Address (street/city/zip)	Home Phone/ Work Phone	Email/Fax
Nancy Taylor, leader	123 West Road Yourtown, CA 00001	(713) 555-0001 (h) (713) 555-0002 (w)	Ntaylor@email.com (713) 555-0003 (fax)
Susan Garrett	6221 Indigo Lane Yourtown, CA 00001	(713) 555-0004 (h) (713) 555-0005 (w)	Sgarrett@email.com
Bob Matthews	254 Jones Road Yourtown, CA 00001	(281) 555-0006 (h) (281) 555-0007 (w)	Bmatthew@email.com

How to Handle Latecomers

- If some miss Orientation, allow them to watch the _Orientation_ video.
- If some miss Orientation **and** the first meeting, allow them to watch the _Orientation_ video and the first section of the _Food Exchange Plan_ video.

Note: Ideally, it is best to set a standard from the beginning that _no one_ will be admitted to the group after the second meeting. Assure any latecomers they are welcome to be a part of First Place, but for their benefit they need to wait for the next Orientation. Help them locate another group in your area, if possible.

The reasons for this recommendation are that the leader would have to repeat introductions and schedules, as well as prepare new rosters and other paperwork; and that the new member (1) may not bond with other members of the group, causing potential problems in sharing personal feelings with the new person; (2) will have questions that have already been answered, thus slowing down the progress of the group; (3) may not have a commitment level as high as it would be had he or she joined the group from the beginning.

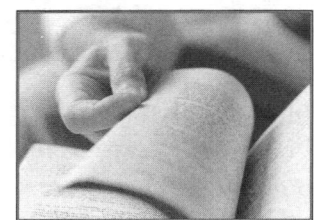

Leadership Guidelines

LEADERSHIP PRINCIPLES

We proclaim him, admonishing and teaching everyone with all wisdom, so that we may present everyone perfect in Christ (Colossians 1:28).

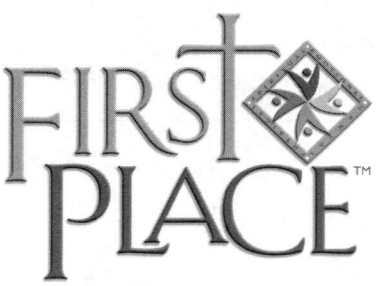

MISSION STATEMENT

The goal of the First Place leader is to lead members to put Jesus Christ in first place in their lives by

- Inspiring them to build godly disciplines into every area of their lives: spiritual, emotional, physical and mental;

- Reviving motivation and instilling hope within each member so that he or she, through the Lord's guidance, can make positive behavioral changes;

- Providing the member with knowledge of the Live-It plan and other healthy lifestyle information.

BUILD OPENNESS AND TRUST

1. Relate with group members in such a way as to build openness and trust in communication.

   Let your conversation be always full of grace, seasoned with salt, so that you may know how to answer everyone (Colossians 4:6).

2. Arrive early, demonstrating your faithfulness to be there for your members.
3. Learn group members' names.
4. Relate personally with individual members through conversations related to previously shared information.
5. Be yourself! Be real!
6. Follow through—if you say you will do something, *do* it!

BUILD FELLOWSHIP AND ACCOUNTABILITY

1. Encourage members to stand in the gap for their fellow group members.

   Carry each other's burdens, and in this way you will fulfill the law of Christ (Galatians 6:2).

2. Cultivate fellowship through icebreakers, prayer partners and discussions.
3. Be persistent in asking stimulating questions that encourage discussion.
4. Have members share testimonies, tips for dealing with obstacles and victories.
5. When sharing prayer requests aloud in class, ask members to share personal needs. Remind them that this is a support group, and in order to support one another, we need to know how to *specifically* pray for one another.

BE COMMITTED AND COMPASSIONATE

1. Demonstrate compassion for and a commitment to your members.

   Therefore, as God's chosen people, holy and dearly loved, clothe yourselves with compassion, kindness, humility, gentleness and patience (Colossians 3:12).

2. Be a good listener.
3. Empathize with members' feelings and show concern.
4. Give members recognition at every possible opportunity.
5. Contact members who miss a meeting and let them know you are concerned about them.

BE PREPARED

1. Teach group members relevant and practical information that will meet their needs.
2. Prepare thoroughly for Bible study and Wellness Worksheet issues.

3. Look like a leader! Wear clothes that fit properly and enhance your appearance.
4. Lead members to set realistic and wise goals that are specific, measurable, attainable, relevant and trackable.
5. Present topics in a clear and orderly manner.
6. Make members aware of First Place materials that are available, such as the newsletter.
7. Use motivational stories, attention getters, guest speakers and group activities that will meet various learning styles.

BE THE LEADER

1. Be the administrator/facilitator of what goes on in the meeting.
2. Make each session your own by using your gifts and abilities to make the meeting unique.
3. Be prepared and prayed up, sensitive to the Holy Spirit and to the needs of the group.
4. Be flexible and willing to change your plans as the Spirit leads.
5. Leave your problems at Jesus' feet, and focus on the needs of your group members during the meeting time. Use leader meetings to express and pray about your burdens and needs.
6. Take control of class discussions, making sure the time is spent wisely. Be prepared to take care of problem people:

A Talker: To prevent one person from dominating discussions, set up guidelines in the first meeting. Communicate with members the importance of allowing everyone the opportunity to share in discussions. **Tip:** *Ask everyone to give one-word or one-sentence answers for some of the questions.*

Dropouts: On occasion people join First Place and later realize they cannot fulfill their commitment. Encourage them to continue, but if they decide to drop out, let them know that you will still consider them part of the group. **Tip:** *Keep lines of communication open through notes or phone calls. It is always important to keep the door open for members to return at a later session.*

A Shy Person: Be sensitive to people in your group who are shy and may feel embarrassed if called on to pray or speak in class. Look for ways to include them in the group. **Tip:** *Small-group or paired activities might help them feel safe and secure.*

Be Positive

1. Positively lead members to godly belief in their own success.

   I can do everything through him who gives me strength (Philippians 4:13).

2. Try to direct all thoughts, comments and discussions toward the positive view. Don't dwell on the negative.
3. Do not condemn or accuse. Show group members the possible consequences of both wise and foolish choices. Focus on the benefits of behavioral changes.
4. Remind members that God is the God of second chances and that one slip doesn't mean all is lost.
5. Lead members to solve their problems practically, without expecting you to have every answer.
6. Be an encourager! Close every meeting with words of hope.

Be Cooperative with Other Leaders

1. Work in loving cooperation with assistants, coleaders and members.

   Make my joy complete by being like-minded, having the same love, being one in spirit and purpose (Philippians 2:2).

2. Work with the team in unity and with one mind. This is a ministry, and you are there to serve one another.
3. Communicate! Have meetings before each First Place session to insure that all is being done to meet the needs of the members in your group.
4. Pray! Pray for the members and those on your leadership team.
5. Always be looking for the potential leader in your assistants and in other group members. This is a great opportunity for mentoring.

SHARING CHRIST THROUGH FIRST PLACE

Do not miss this great opportunity to share the story of Jesus Christ. Take time to give your testimony, or to ask a member to share his or her testimony. After the testimony, tell the group that you will be available to speak with anyone who may have questions regarding their salvation. Be prepared, with the help of the Holy Spirit, to lead an unsaved member to faith in Jesus Christ.

Share the following Steps to Becoming a Christian (also found in the *First Place Member's Guide*). After a member receives Christ, give him or her a copy of Steps to Spiritual Growth (pp. 91-92 of this *Leader's Guide*).

STEPS TO BECOMING A CHRISTIAN

THE BIBLE SAYS

- We were made for God.
- God seeks a relationship with each of us.
- God yearns for us to spend eternity with Him in heaven.

THE BAD NEWS

Sin separates us from God and eliminates our hope for heaven. Sin means missing what God wants for our lives. Think of a bull's-eye and arrows that have missed the center mark; sin means missing God's mark for us.

THE GOOD NEWS

- Jesus, God's only Son, came to Earth in the form of a human.
- He willingly became our sacrifice by dying on the cross for our sins.
- We cannot save ourselves. Jesus' blood covers all our sins and reconciles us to God.

➣ Have you ever made the decision to ask Jesus Christ to be your Savior? ☐ yes   ☐ no

If you answered yes, on a separate sheet of paper write about your personal experience.
If your answer is no, please open your heart to God now. These are the simple steps to take:

- **Acknowledge that you are a sinner.** "For all have sinned and fall short of the glory of God" (Romans 3:23).
- **Acknowledge that sin separates you from God.** "For the wages of sin is death, but the gift of God is eternal life in Christ Jesus our Lord" (Romans 6:23).
- **Acknowledge that Christ died for you.** "But God demonstrates his own love for us in this: While we were still sinners, Christ died for us" (Romans 5:8).
- **Receive Christ as Savior.** "If you confess with your mouth 'Jesus is Lord,' and believe in your heart that God raised him from the dead, you will be saved. For it is with your heart that you believe and are justified, and it is with your mouth that you confess and are saved" (Romans 10:9-10).

Now pray these words:

Dear God,
I know I am a sinner and separated from You. I believe You love me and that You sent Jesus to die on the cross for me. I accept You as my Savior and my Lord. Please forgive me of my sin and teach me how to give You first place in my life. Amen.

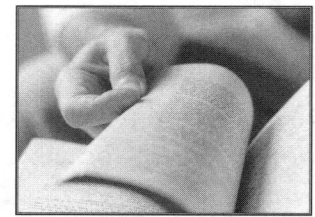

Leadership Preparation

BUILDING YOUR WEEKLY MEETING LESSON PLANS

Every session will begin with teaching the Live-It Plan and the Commitment Record. However, for the next 10 weeks you will teach a different lesson each week. The class structure goes as follows:

15 minutes—Greet and weigh members

20 minutes—Wellness Spotlight

30 minutes—Bible study

+10 minutes—Prayer time

75 minutes (1 hour, 15 minutes) total

Greet and Weigh Members

Arrive early and prepare for the lesson before members arrive. Have an assistant weigh members as you greet other members. For Weigh-In Guidelines, see page 87.

Wellness Spotlight

Each Wellness Worksheet (in the Bible studies) or Essential Wellness Worksheet (in the *Member's Guide*) is packed with information to use during this 20-minute period. In fact, you can't use them all. You can pick what will work for your group. The Weekly Meeting Plans beginning on page 00 are intended for a group of first-time members. If you lead a group that has been meeting together for a while, you can use the Wellness Worksheets in the Bible studies instead of those suggested in the plans.

BIBLE STUDY

A Leader's Discussion Guide is included in the back of each Bible study. You will use this guide to build the lessons. Remember that Bible study time is meant to be a discussion. Try not to lecture. Stimulate discussions by asking open-end questions. Be cautious not to contribute too much, but try instead to draw out members in discussion.

PRAYER TIME

It is difficult to keep from spending so much time during the Wellness Spotlight and Bible study that you might go overtime and neglect the prayer time. Group prayer time is essential to growth and bonding among the members. Be aware of the time, and close the Bible study with plenty of time for prayer.

YOUR TIME, THEIR TIME

Time is important to everyone. We need time to spend time alone with God, with our families, at work and in church activities. Meetings that often go overtime will frustrate many, and by the end of the meeting, they might not be paying attention because they are too busy thinking of what they could—or should—be doing instead. Be sensitive to others by dismissing the meeting on time.

LESSON PLAN

The time it takes to plan each lesson is time worth spending. It allows you to arrive prepared and with everything you need. The Weekly Lesson Plan Form on pages 00-00 will aid you in planning for the weekly meeting.

HOW TO USE THE WORKSHEETS

The worksheets are found in the *First Place Member's Guide* and the Bible studies. Their purpose is to inform members about important health, fitness and spiritual issues. The following descriptions will help you understand the use of the worksheets.

WELLNESS WORKSHEETS

- Prepared by Jody Wilkinson, M.D. and found in the Bible studies
- Contain helpful information in the spiritual, emotional, physical and mental areas
- Designed to be interactive and may be completed by members individually or during meetings

ESSENTIAL WELLNESS WORKSHEETS

- Needed by every member during the first session (see Weekly Meeting Plans, pp. 38-73)
- Discussed during the Wellness Spotlight portion of each meeting

ADDITIONAL WORKSHEETS

- Found in the *First Place Member's Guide*
- May be used as Extra Mile assignments which are not usually discussed during the group meeting (also may be used if the group has a special need)
- May be used at the leader's discretion or for further study

THINGS TO REMEMBER

1. The Session Overview (pp. 38-39) suggests when each essential Wellness Worksheet should be presented.
2. The Wellness Spotlight is the time set aside to discuss the Wellness Worksheet.
3. Allow 10 to 20 minutes each week for the Wellness Spotlight.
4. You will find an abundance of Wellness Worksheets that allows for more flexibility in meeting the needs of members. For example, after assessing the member surveys, you might find that most members are interested in exercise. You might then choose Wellness Worksheets that focus on exercise for group discussion.
5. Involve members by asking them to facilitate the Wellness Spotlight.
6. Spotlight assignments will be discussed during the following meeting.
7. At-home assignments are located at the end of each Group Meeting Plan. They include Spotlight (SL) and Extra Mile (EM) assignments.
8. The Extra Mile assignments provide information for members who desire further study. Extra Mile assignments are strictly optional and no planned discussion is required.

HOW TO EVALUATE COMMITMENT RECORDS (CRS)

THE GOALS OF EVALUATING A CR

- Accountability
- Encouragement
- Progress tracking

HOW TO EVALUATE CRs OF NEW MEMBERS

- Check for accuracy of food exchanges—for example, if one egg was not counted as one meat and one-half fat, make necessary corrections.
- Check total daily exchanges: Are they within guidelines?
- Check weekly progress.
- Place stickers on CRs for encouragement. Stickers may be found at teacher-supply stores, supermarkets, discount stores, craft stores and Christian bookstores.

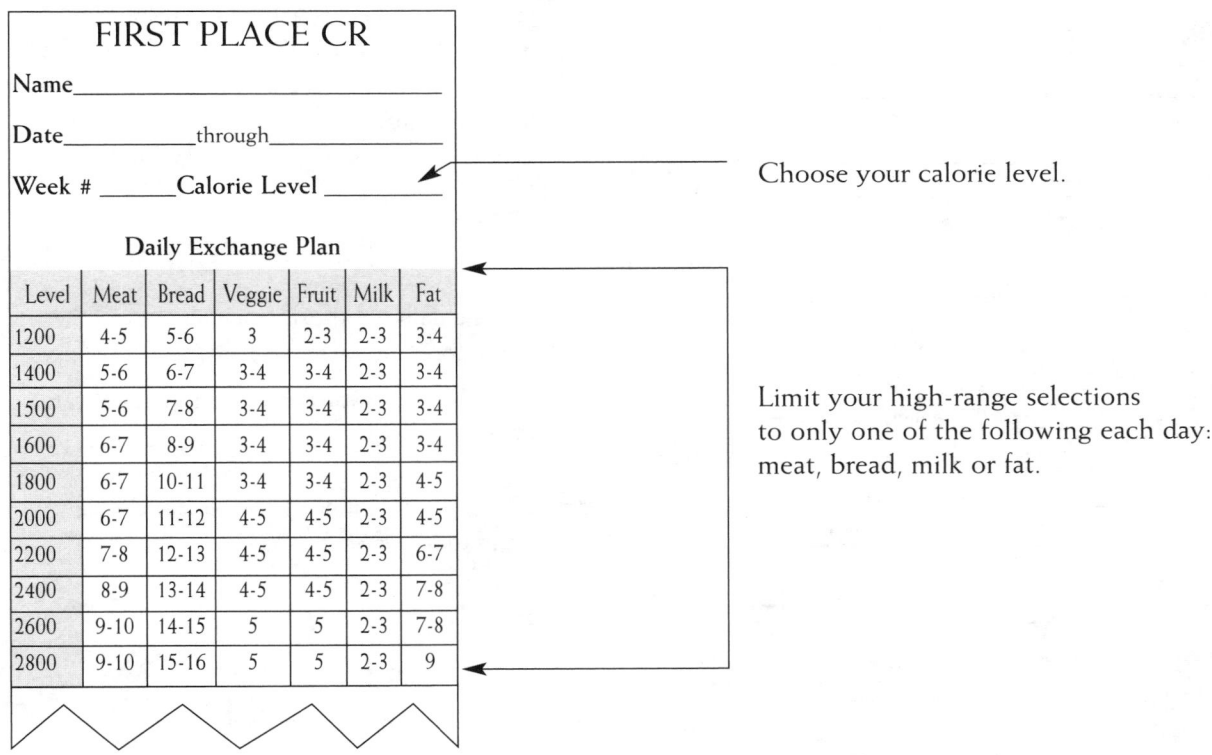

FIRST PLACE CR

Name_____

Date_____through_____

Week # _____Calorie Level _____

Choose your calorie level.

Daily Exchange Plan

Level	Meat	Bread	Veggie	Fruit	Milk	Fat
1200	4-5	5-6	3	2-3	2-3	3-4
1400	5-6	6-7	3-4	3-4	2-3	3-4
1500	5-6	7-8	3-4	3-4	2-3	3-4
1600	6-7	8-9	3-4	3-4	2-3	3-4
1800	6-7	10-11	3-4	3-4	2-3	4-5
2000	6-7	11-12	4-5	4-5	2-3	4-5
2200	7-8	12-13	4-5	4-5	2-3	6-7
2400	8-9	13-14	4-5	4-5	2-3	7-8
2600	9-10	14-15	5	5	2-3	7-8
2800	9-10	15-16	5	5	2-3	9

Limit your high-range selections to only one of the following each day: meat, bread, milk or fat.

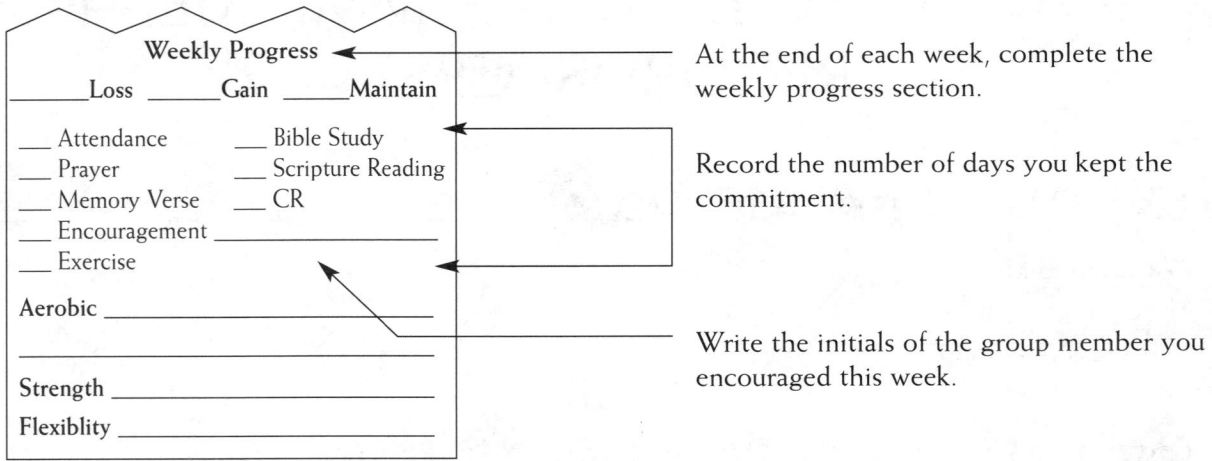

Weekly Progress

_____Loss _____Gain _____Maintain

___ Attendance   ___ Bible Study
___ Prayer   ___ Scripture Reading
___ Memory Verse   ___ CR
___ Encouragement _____
___ Exercise

Aerobic _____

_____

Strength _____

Flexiblity _____

At the end of each week, complete the weekly progress section.

Record the number of days you kept the commitment.

Write the initials of the group member you encouraged this week.

DAY 7:   Date _____

Morning _____

_____

Midday _____

_____

Evening _____

_____

Snacks _____

_____

_____

___ Meat _____	☐ Prayer
___ Bread _____	☐ Bible Study
___ Vegetable ____	☐ Scripture Reading
___ Fruit _____	☐ Memory Verse
___ Milk _____	☐ Encouragement
___ Fat _____	☐ Water_____

Exercise:

Aerobic _____

_____

Strength _____

Flexibility _____

List the foods you have eaten. On this condensed CR it is not necessary to exchange each food choice. It will be the responsibility of each member that the tally marks you list below are accurate regarding each food choice. If you are unsure of an exchange, check the Live-It section of your Member's Guide.

List the daily food-exchange choices to the left of the food groups.

Use tally marks for the actual food and water consumed.

Check off commitments completed. Use tally marks to record each 8-ounce serving of water.

List type and duration of exercise.

FIRST PLACE COMMITMENT RECORD

Name _Kay Smith_

Date _3-19-01_ through _3-25-01_

Memory Verse _Matthew 6:33_

But seek first his kingdom, and his righteousness, and all these things will be given to you as well.

Week # _3_   Calorie Level _1400_

Daily Exchanges

Meat _5-6_   Bread _6-7_   Vegetable _3-4_

Fruit _3-4_   Milk _3-4_   Fat _2-3_

Water _8_

© 2001 First Place

Weekly Progress

Weight Management

Loss _-2 lbs._   Gain _____   Maintain _____

Commitments

✓	Attendance	_6_	Bible Study
_7_	Prayer	_6_	Scripture Reading
_7_	Memory Verse	_7_	CR
✓	Encouragement:	_CR / EE_	

Exercise Aerobic _3 mile walk/30 minute bike ride_

Strength _15 minutes lower body_

Flexibility _____

Comments _Better week! Used CD to walk. Took time to plan before grocery shopping._

Prayer Requests 1) _Pain in my foot_

2) _Joe's yearly check-up Wednesday_

3) _Stress with my job!_

DAY 1 / DATE

Morning _½ cup oatmeal = 1 bread; 1 sl, ww = 1 bread; 8 oz, skim = 1 milk; 1 tb. raisins = ½ fruit; ¼ cup apple juice in oatmeal = ½ fruit_

Midday _cheese broccoli soup = 1 mt; ½ bd/ ½ milk/ ½ fat; 1 oz. lean ham = 1 mt; 2 sl. diet brd = 1 brd; 1 c. tomato = 1 veg; ⅛ avocado = 1 fat_

Evening _4 oz. baked fish = 4 meat; 1 t. mayo light on fish = 1 fat; ½ c. peas = 1 brd; ½ c. corn = 1 brd; ½ c. mushroms, ½ c. cooked onion = 2 veg._

Snacks _4 apricots = 1 fruit; ½ grapefruit = 1 fruit_

7	Meat	////||
6	Bread	////|
4	Vegetable	////
3	Fruit	///
2	Milk	//
3	Fat	///

✓	Prayer
✓	Bible Study
✓	Scripture Reading
✓	Memory Verse
✓	Encouragement
	Water //// ///

Exercise

Aerobic _3 mile walk_

Strength _____

Flexibility _10 min. stretches_

This is a sample of a completed full-sized CR available in packages of 13 pocket-sized forms. One package is included in each Member Kit. Additional packages may be purchased separately.

How to Evaluate Alumni CRs

- Check the weekly progress section of the CR.
- If there is a gain or an extreme loss, evaluate the CR as you would for a new member.
- Check other commitments and give praise where progress is shown. Provide encouragement where improvement is needed.
- Where lengthy comments are needed, use Post-it Notes.

Things to Remember

- Always be encouraging, pointing out mistakes in a positive manner.
- If you sense discouragement or lack of commitment, make a personal contact.
- It is important to evaluate CRs promptly and return them at the next meeting.
- Alumni who have reached their goal have the option of not filling out the CR, however, many successful members have maintained their weight loss by continuing the accountability practice of filling out the CR.

CREATIVE IDEAS

The following ideas are provided to give you alternatives to the suggested meeting plans or to provide activities for groups made up of members who have been in First Place groups for awhile.

FOOD BANK FOOD RAISER

Each member brings an amount of nonperishable packaged or canned food to class equal to the amount of weight he or she has lost. Members are often amazed at the difficulty of carrying that amount of weight. Donate the food to a local food pantry.

FOOD CRITICS CORNER

Have each member find and research one restaurant in your area—you might want to assign them one. Have them evaluate the menu to see if it can be considered a First Place restaurant. Examples could be 1 star = poor, 2 stars = fair, 3 stars = good, 4 stars = excellent and 5 stars = superior. Have members explain how they came to their evaluations.

POUND-O-FAT

Buy a pound of fat from your local butcher and put it in a clear plastic bag. Pass it around and let everyone see the importance of losing even one pound.

BOOK FAIR

Ask each member to bring a recipe book or any other book that has helped him or her keep the First Place commitments. Have each person briefly share how the book has helped him or her with the First Place program. Books should be motivational and pertaining to one or more of the four areas of First Place: spiritual, emotional, physical and mental.

MEASURING MISHAPS

Bring a food scale and measuring cups to the meeting along with several foods that are often measured incorrectly, such as baked potatoes, meat, cheese, butter, mayonnaise, etc. Let members estimate one exchange without measuring it. Then measure the food to find the true measurement. This will encourage members to measure food properly.

THE HUMAN YO-YO

Provide a balloon for each member. Ask members to blow up balloons and let the air out several times. Call to their attention how much easier the balloon was to blow up each time, and how much larger it got each time. Compare this to the weight cycling or yo-yo syndrome of gaining and losing and gaining and losing. Suggest that members keep the balloons as reminders.

The Harvest

In a spring session bring a package of fast-growing seeds, a package of soil and medium-sized paper cups to class. Set up a table where group members can plant their seeds in the paper cups. If necessary, provide directions for planting (see seed package). Begin the meeting by asking members what is necessary for the growth of this plant. Use the analogy that our spiritual lives are dependent on necessary components as well. Have the group use a concordance and do a word study on the words "grow," "growth" or "growing" in the Bible. Challenge members to nurture their plants and bring them to the Victory Celebration.

Dining Out Field Trip

Meet at a restaurant instead of the usual meeting place. Go over the Eating-on-the-Go Guidelines in the *Member's Guide* and discuss them as you look over the menu and during the meal. Bring a scale, measuring cups and spoons for added fun!

Supermarket Savvy

Many grocery chains have people who give healthy heart shopping tours. This is a wonderful field trip if available in your area. If such a tour is not available, you can have a meeting that focuses on grocery planning and reading labels. Fill out a grocery list based on a few meals from your two weeks of menu plans.

Exercise Commitment

Invite a fitness professional such as an aerobic instructor or personal trainer and let him or her do the talking. You can even turn the class into an aerobics class or a meeting at the gym. Instruct members to wear appropriate exercise clothing.

Professional Image Class

Call around to boutique-type apparel stores and ask if they have someone who can talk about fashion. Ask if they have any special knowledge of helping people look their best. A makeover is always fun (even for men). See if there is someone available who can do hair and makeup as well.

Out with the Old, In with the Recycled!

After the meeting, have a clothes swap. Many groups like to trade clothes as they lose weight. In this way, members can have a few new clothes as they work toward their goals.

Salad Luncheon or Dinner

This is a great way to celebrate success midway through a session. Everyone brings two cups of salad items and something to drink. Assign these items the week before. The leader could provide bowls, napkins and forks. Serve 15 minutes before the meeting starts and allow members a few minutes of meeting time to finish their salads.

Baked Potato Supper

Another great way to celebrate is with a potato supper. Have each member sign up to bring a healthy potato topping. You provide the baked potatoes.

VICTORY CELEBRATION SUGGESTIONS

A Victory Celebration is held at the end of each 13-week session. The following suggestions are provided to get you started, but let these ideas spark your own creativity.

A Victory Dinner or Luncheon

Food may be prepared in your church kitchen, catered or provided by members. If you have First Place funds available, you may want to provide the drinks and paper goods.

Decorations

Ask for volunteers to help make decorations and do the decorating. You might want to decorate with a First Place theme. Use First Place mugs as vases. Fill them with fresh flowers and give them as rewards for leaders, assistants or group members. Tape measures make fun napkin rings: cut a tape measure at 6-inch intervals and glue the ends together to make rings. Another idea is to decorate with a holiday theme, depending on the time of year.

Style Show

Call members who have had a noticeable weight loss. Ask them to model something they wore before they lost weight. After the style show, models change into properly fitting clothes and read their testimonies about how much weight they have lost and what First Place has meant to them.

Special Speaker

Invite a speaker who will present an educational or motivational message. The message could relate to any of the four areas of personal development covered in First Place. **Caution**: It is a good idea to use speakers you have heard before.

Skits

Present a skit. Ask volunteers from your group to develop and perform a skit on behavior modification, eating out or spiritual growth.

Awards Time

Recognize each member's accomplishments. Present awards such as "Most Consistent First Place Member," "Exercise Award," "Live-It Expert," "Neatest Commitment Record," "Prayer Warrior," "Reached Goal Weight," or any other creative award. Be sure to give an award to each member. Consider special accomplishments, such as a diabetic who was faithful to a program to control blood sugar or a member who lowered his or her cholesterol. Successes in all areas should be recognized. The greatest victory of all would be if a member accepted Jesus during the session. This would certainly constitute a very special recognition. Be sensitive to those members who are shy. Recognition should be done with respect for the individual's feelings.

TESTIMONY TIME

Invite members to give testimony about changes God has helped them to accomplish through First Place. This is a special blessing. Plan these testimonies before the victory celebration. Give volunteers a five-minute time limit for their testimonies.

MUSIC

Ask someone in your group to provide special music.

BE CREATIVE

Be on the lookout for different options for your Victory Celebration. Network with other First Place groups in your area for ideas. You might collaborate with area First Place groups for a victory rally to multiply the ministry and get the word out about First Place.

VISITORS

Victory Celebrations are a great time to bring guests who might be interested in joining First Place.

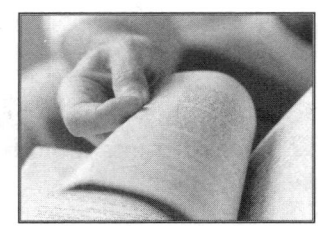

Weekly Meeting Plans

SESSION OVERVIEW

Week #	Learning Activities	At-Home Assignments
Week 1	Get Acquainted Understand the Live-It Plan How to Use a CR	*SL: Finding Your Healthy Weight Choosing a Calorie Level **EM: Establishing a Quiet Time
Week 2	Determine Healthy Weight and Weight Loss Goals Review Live-It Plan and CR Commit to Quiet Time	SL: Understanding the Nutrition Facts Panel EM: First Place Physical Activity Program The Activity Pyramid
Week 3	Understanding the Nutrition Facts Panel Discuss Week One Bible Study	SL: What's the Big Deal About Water? Hiding God's Word in Your Heart EM: Understanding Weight Gain and Obesity—Part I
Week 4	What's the Big Deal About Water? Hiding God's Word in Your Heart Discuss Week Two Bible Study	SL: Eating Habits Inventory EM: Understanding Weight Gain and Obesity—Part II
Week 5	Eating Habits Inventory Discuss Week Three Bible Study	SL: Preventing Osteoporosis EM: Starting a Walking Program How Physically Active Are You?
Week 6	Preventing Osteoporosis Discuss Week Four Bible Study	SL: Changing Recipes Calculating Exchanges for a Recipe EM: Understanding Weight Gain and Obesity—Part III A Flexible Fitness Program

*SL means Spotlight and refers to the essential worksheets found in the *Member's Guide*, containing information every first-time member needs in order to better understand the First Place program. They are meant to be discussed during the Wellness Spotlight section of the meeting.

**EM refers to the Extra Mile worksheets that are intended for members' information only. However, any Extra Mile worksheet might be discussed during a meeting if the need arises.

Week #	Learning Activities	At-Home Assignments
Week 7	Changing Recipes Calculating Exchanges for a Recipe Discuss Week Five Bible Study	SL: The Anytime, Anywhere Restaurant Guide EM: Testing Your Health-Related Fitness Monitoring Your Exercise Intensity
Week 8	The Anytime, Anywhere Restaurant Guide Discuss Week Six Bible Study	SL: Sugar—Sweetness by Any Other Name EM: Fitting in Strength Training Bible Study Wellness Worksheet
Week 9	Sugar—Sweetness by Any Other Name Discuss Week Seven Bible Study	SL: The Truth About Fats EM: Running Your Way to Health and Fitness Bible Study Wellness Worksheet
Week 10	The Truth About Fats Discuss Week Eight Bible Study	SL: Choosing High-Fiber Foods Meatless Meals EM: Bicycling Your Way to Health and Fitness
Week 11	Choosing High-Fiber Foods Meatless Meals Discuss Week Nine Bible Study	SL: Off to a Good Start Sharing Your Faith EM: Water Exercise for Health and Fitness
Week 12	Off to a Good Start Sharing Your Faith Discuss Week Ten Bible Study	SL: Write personal testimony using Sharing Your Faith
Week 13	Sharing Your Testimony Victory Celebration	

13 WEEKLY MEETING PLANS

GROUP MEETING WEEK ONE

LEARNING ACTIVITIES	AT-HOME ASSIGNMENTS
Get Acquainted *Understand the Live-It Plan* *How to Use a CR*	*SL: Finding Your Healthy Weight* *Choosing a Calorie Level* *EM: Establishing a Quiet Time*

BEFORE THE MEETING

1. Review the steps to Getting Started (pp. 10-18) and preview the Live-It segment of the *Food Exchange Plan* video. Consider extending the length of this first meeting by 15 to 30 minutes.

2. Prayerfully approach the responsibility of leading a First Place group. Ask for God's wisdom as you follow His direction in leading your group. Pray Hebrews 10:24 for yourself—that you would be able to spur group members on to love and good deeds. Then pray for each member by name.

3. Meet with your assistant to prepare.

    a. Pray together.

    b. Discuss the Weigh-In Guidelines (p. 87) and have assistant fill out the Weigh-In Chart (pp. 85-86) with members' names.

    c. Make a copy of the First Place Group Roster (p. 84).

    d. Make copies of the Prayer Partner Request Form (p. 90) to give to each member. You will need a basket or a similar container for members to place their Prayer Request Forms in at the beginning of the meeting. At the end of the meeting, each member will draw a request from the container and pray for that request during the week.

    e. Select someone to take "before" pictures of each member at the first meeting. Keep these pictures until the final session to help members see their progress.

    f. Make name tags for everyone in the group. You might consider making permanent name tags.

4. Call members to remind them of day, time and location of the meeting. Ask them to fill out the Member Survey (p. 88) ahead of time and turn it in at the first meeting. Have additional Member Surveys at the first meeting for those who forget theirs.

a. If child care will be available, check with each member to learn how many children will be coming and the children's ages.

b. If you choose to extend the length of this first meeting, inform members ahead of time.

5. Arrive early to set up the meeting room with chairs in a semicircle and at least one table for the name tags, roster and Prayer Partner Request Form container.

a. Set up the TV and VCR, and cue the video so that it is ready for viewing during the meeting.

b. Place a Prayer Partner Request Form on each chair.

c. Have extra pens or pencils, paper and Bibles available for those who might have forgotten them.

THE MEETING

1. **Arrival Activity—15 Minutes**

   a. Greet members.

   b. Place the Group Roster on a table with the name tags and instruct members to check it for accuracy and make corrections if necessary.

   c. Privately weigh each member and record weights on the Weigh-In Chart.

   d. Take "before" pictures (optional).

   e. Collect Member Surveys.

   f. Direct members to complete the Prayer Partner Request Forms and place them in the container provided.

2. **Opening—20 Minutes**

   a. Open with prayer.

   b. Ask group members to introduce themselves. Keep this brief and plan a get acquainted activity for the second meeting.

   c. Briefly review the *Nine Commitments* video.

3. **Wellness Spotlight—20 Minutes**

   a. Watch the Live-It segment of the *Food Exchange Plan* video.

   • Assure members that they don't need to remember everything on the video. Suggest that they read the *Member's Guide* "Live-It Plan" for further instruction.

   b. Inform members that they will begin to fill out the CRs this first week. Reassure them that this is a learning experience and that perfection is not the goal.

4. **Question and Answer Time—10 Minutes**

5. **At-Home Assignments—10 Minutes**

Note: Leaders may vary the method of presenting at-home assignments for each week according to available time. Suggestions:

- Assign them verbally.

- List them on a chalkboard or white board.

- Write them out, photocopy and give each member a copy at the end of the meeting.

a. Instruct members to fill out their CRs to the best of their ability, striving to keep all of the commitments. (Exception: the Bible study begins after the second meeting.)

b. Remind members that the two-week menu plans are included in the Bible study. Using these menu choices will help them learn exchanges and will enable them to fill out the CR with ease.

c. Assign members a Scripture verse to memorize this week.

d. Distribute the Wellness Worksheets. Explain the difference between Spotlight (SL) and Extra Mile (EM) assignments.

- Finding Your Healthy Weight (pp. 34-36, MG***)

- Choosing a Calorie Level (pp. 37-39, MG)

- Establishing a Quiet Time (pp. 13-14, MG)

e. After completing the Wellness Worksheets, encourage members to prayerfully consider their weight-loss goals (which should be no more than two pounds per week).

6. **Prayer Time—5 Minutes**

a. Ask members to select a Prayer Partner Request Form.

b. Close in prayer with members holding hands in a circle.

AFTER THE MEETING

1. Complete a new Group Roster, incorporating any corrections, and photocopy it to hand out at next week's meeting.

2. Call members to see if they have questions concerning the Live-It Plan (pp. 31-73, MG).

3. Check for accuracy on the Weigh-In Chart.

4. Contact absentee members, and arrange a time for them to watch the *Food Exchange Plan* video.

***MG denotes *Member's Guide* page numbers.

GROUP MEETING WEEK TWO

LEARNING ACTIVITIES	AT-HOME ASSIGNMENTS
Determine Healthy Weight and Weight-Loss Goals *Review Live-It Plan and CR* *Establishing a Quiet Time*	*SL: Understanding the Nutrition Facts Panel* *EM: First Place Physical Activity Program* *The Activity Pyramid*

BEFORE THE MEETING

1. Review the Live-It segment of the *Food Exchange Plan* video.
2. Review the Wellness Worksheets and highlight or make a list of the points you plan to emphasize.
    a. Finding Your Healthy Weight (pp. 34-36, MG)
    b. Choosing a Calorie Level (pp. 37-39, MG)
    c. Establishing a Quiet Time (pp. 13-14, MG)
3. Call members and ask if they have any questions about the Live-It Plan or filling out the CR.
4. Pray for group members.
5. Purchase stickers for encouragement to place on CRs and stars to reward those who recite the Scripture memory verse.
6. Make copies of the group roster for each member.
7. Arrive early to set up the room.
    a. Set up the TV and VCR, and cue the video so that it is ready for viewing during the meeting.
    b. Place a Group Roster and a Prayer Partner Request Form on each chair.
    c. Have extra pens or pencils, paper and Bibles available for those who might have forgotten them.

THE MEETING

1. **Arrival Activity—15 Minutes**
    a. Greet members and have name tags sitting out for members when they arrive.
    b. Weigh members, record weights and listen to Scripture memory verse recitations.
    d. Collect members' completed CRs.
    e. Direct members to complete new Prayer Partner Request Forms and place them in the container.

2. **Opening—10 Minutes**

   a. Open with prayer.

   b. Begin with one or more of the following icebreaker activities:

   1) Ask members to introduce themselves and tell about their jobs, families and hobbies.

   2) Ask members to share what they hope to learn/accomplish during the next 11 weeks.

   3) Ask each member to go to another member, preferably someone he or she doesn't know and touch fingertips. Then give them one minute to share an unknown fact about themselves.

3. **Wellness Spotlight—30 Minutes**

   a. View the second segment of the *Food Exchange Plan* video.

   b. Ask members to complete the cover page of CR for week two. Help members fill in the Daily Exchanges according to their calorie levels.

   c. Remind members that they should begin their CRs with their next meal.

   d. Allow time for questions regarding the Live-It Plan.

4. **Review the Wellness Worksheets—10 Minutes**

   a. Finding Your Healthy Weight

   1) Briefly go through the steps using specific examples.

   2) Discuss questions or concerns over weight-loss goals.

   b. Choosing a Calorie Level

   1) Stress the importance of eating the proper amounts and exchanges.

   2) Caution women to eat no less than 1400 calories and men to eat no less than 1500 calories.

   c. Establishing a Quiet Time

   Encourage members to write their prayers in their prayer journal each day.

6. **At-Home Assignments**

   Instruct members to complete the following assignments before the next meeting:

   a. Complete each daily assignment in week one of the Bible study.

   b. Read and complete the Wellness Worksheets.

   1) Understanding the Nutrition Facts Panel (pp. 132-134, MG)

   2) Physical Activity Program (pp. 74-78, MG)

   3) The Activity Pyramid (pp. 79-81, MG)

   c. Memorize this week's Scripture memory verse.

   d. Encourage one other group member.

   e. Complete the CR.

7. **Prayer Time—10 Minutes**

   a. Discuss with members that prayer requests must be kept confidential.

   b. Invite members to share their personal prayer requests and then direct the prayer time by asking questions that require personal responses. For example: "What is something that makes putting Christ first in your life a struggle?"

   c. Instruct members to record requests on the Group Prayer Requests page at the end week one in the Bible study.

   d. Have each member select a Prayer Partner Request Form from the container.

   e. Join hands in a circle. Suggest that all members pray silently for God to guide them in a more Christ-centered life.

   f. Ask for a volunteer to close in prayer.

AFTER THE MEETING

1. Evaluate members' CRs. Remember to be positive with any comments. (Refer to How to Evaluate CRs on pages 29-32 for help.)
2. Record each member's weight-loss goal on the Weigh-In Chart.
3. Calculate weight loss for each member, and determine the group total for the week.
4. Contact absentees by phone or a note, encouraging them to attend next week and informing them of the At-Home Assignments for the week.

GROUP MEETING WEEK THREE

LEARNING ACTIVITIES	AT-HOME ASSIGNMENTS
Understanding the Nutrition Facts Panel *Discussion of week one of the Bible study*	*SL: What's the Big Deal About Water?* *Hiding God's Word in Your Heart* *EM: Understanding Weight Gain and Obesity—* *Part I*

BEFORE THE MEETING

1. Review the Wellness Worksheet: Understanding the Nutrition Facts Panel (pp. 132-134, MG) and highlight or make a list of the points you plan to emphasize.

   • Collect sample products with Nutritional Facts Panels on them to use in meeting.

2. Complete week one of the Bible study.
   Use the leader's guide at the back of the Bible study to prepare a discussion.

3. Memorize the Scripture memory verse.

4. Arrive early to set up the room.

   a. Set up chairs and tables.

   b. Place a Prayer Partner Request Form on each chair.

   c. Have extra pens or pencils, paper and Bibles available for those who might have forgotten them.

THE MEETING

1. **Arrival Activity—15 Minutes**

   a. Greet and encourage each member.

   b. Weigh members, record weights and listen to Scripture memory verse recitations.

   c. Collect the CRs and return the evaluated ones.

   d. Direct members to complete new Prayer Request Forms and place them in the container.

   e. Open in prayer.

   f. **Option:** View the *Nine Commitments* video segment as members are arriving and weighing in.

2. **Wellness Spotlight—15 Minutes**

   Discuss the Wellness Worksheet: Understanding the Nutritional Facts Panel:

   a. Invite members to look at the examples on the worksheet.

   b. Discuss the ingredients list, noting that the ingredients are listed in descending order of the amounts.

   c. **Optional**: Hand out the examples you collected. Group members could work in teams to discuss the labels, depending on the size of the group.

   d. Give members a few seconds to evaluate the information.

   e. Allow each team or member to report to the group how that product would be listed on the CR.

3. **Bible Study—30 Minutes**

   Facilitate a discussion of week one of the Bible study.

4. **At-Home Assignments**

   Instruct members to complete the following assignments before the next meeting:

   a. Complete week two of the Bible study.

   b. Read and complete the Wellness Worksheets.

      1) What's the Big Deal About Water? (pp. 129-131, MG)

      2) Hiding God's Word in Your Heart (pp. 23-25, MG)

      3) Understanding Weight Gain and Obesity—Part I (pp. 111-114, MG)

   c. Memorize this week's Scripture memory verse.

   d. Encourage one other group member.

   e. Complete the CR.

5. **Prayer Time—10 Minutes**

   a. Instruct members to record requests on the Group Prayer Request Form at the end of week two in the Bible study.

   b. Have each member select a Prayer Partner Request Form from the container.

   c. Close in prayer.

AFTER THE MEETING

1. Evaluate members' CRs.
2. Calculate weight loss for each member, and determine the group total for the week.
3. Contact absentees by phone or note, encouraging them to attend next week and informing them of the At-Home Assignments for the week.

GROUP MEETING WEEK FOUR

LEARNING ACTIVITIES	AT-HOME ASSIGNMENTS
What's the Big Deal About Water?	*SL: Eating Habits Inventory*
Hiding God's Word in Your Heart	*EM: Understanding Weight Gain and Obesity—*
Discussion of week two of the Bible study	*Part II*

BEFORE THE MEETING

1. Review the Wellness Worksheets and highlight or make a list of the points you plan to emphasize.
   a. What's the Big Deal About Water? (pp. 129-131, MG)
   b. Hiding God's Word in Your Heart (pp. 23-25, MG)
2. Complete week two of the Bible study.
   Use the leader's guide at the back of the Bible study to prepare a discussion.
3. Memorize the Scripture memory verse.
4. Arrive early to set up the room.
   a. Set up chairs and tables.
   b. Place a Prayer Partner Request Form on each chair.
   c. Have extra pens or pencils, paper and Bibles available for those who might have forgotten them.

THE MEETING

1. **Arrival Activity—15 Minutes**
   a. Greet and encourage each member.
   b. Weigh members, record weights and listen to Scripture memory verse recitations.
   c. Collect the CRs and return the evaluated ones.
   d. Direct members to complete new Prayer Partner Request Forms and place them in the container.
   e. Open in prayer.
   f. **Optional:** View the *Nine Commitments* video segment as members are arriving and weighing in.
2. **Wellness Spotlight—20 Minutes**
   Discuss the Wellness Worksheets.
   a. What's the Big Deal About Water?

1) Ask how many are drinking eight glasses of water a day.

2) Encourage those who aren't drinking enough water to add a glass each day until they are drinking eight glasses of water per day.

b. Hiding God's Word in Your Heart

1) Encourage members to think of a way to remember the reference—for example, a person might say "I have two teenagers, 15 and 13. They're always roaming around" to remember Romans 15:13. Funny or real-life word pictures can be used to spark memories.

2) Once they've come up with a word picture, have members attach the first word or phrase to the reference so they can be remembered together—for example, Romans 15:13 starts out "May the God of hope," so a member might say "Anyone with teenagers 15 and 13 needs the God of hope."

3) Help members learn the verse by breaking it into several phrases.

4) Finish by playing the Scripture memory song on the CD.

5) Apply the tips on "How to Memorize Scripture" to next week's Scripture memory verse.

6) Encourage members to learn all 10 of the Scripture memory verses and ask for two volunteers to quote the first two memory verses from weeks one and two.

3. **Bible Study—30 Minutes**

Facilitate a discussion of week two of the Bible study.

4. **At-Home Assignments**

Instruct members to complete the following assignments before the next meeting:

a. Complete week three of the Bible study.

b. Read and complete the Wellness Worksheets.

1) Understanding Your Eating Habits (pp. 121-128, MG)

2) Understanding Weight Gain and Obesity—Part II (pp. 115-117, MG)

c. Memorize this week's Scripture memory verse.

d. Encourage one other group member.

e. Complete the CR.

5. **Prayer Time—10 Minutes**

a. Ask for prayer requests and praises. Remind members to record requests on the Group Prayer Requests page at the end of week three in the Bible study.

b. Have each member select a Prayer Partner Request Form from the container.

c. Close in prayer.

AFTER THE MEETING

1. Evaluate members' CRs.
2. Calculate weight loss for each member and determine the group total for the week.
3. Contact absentees by phone or note, encouraging them to attend next week and informing them of the At-Home Assignments for the week.

GROUP MEETING WEEK FIVE

LEARNING ACTIVITIES	AT-HOME ASSIGNMENTS
Eating Habits Inventory *Discussion of week three of the Bible study*	*SL: Preventing Osteoporosis* *Starting a Walking Program* *EM: How Physically Active Are You?*

BEFORE THE MEETING

1. Review the Wellness Worksheet: Understanding Your Eating Habits (pp. 121-128, *MG*) and highlight or make a list of the points you plan to emphasize.
2. Complete week three of the Bible study.
   Use the leader's guide at the back of the Bible study to prepare a discussion.
3. Memorize the Scripture memory verse.
4. Arrive early to set up the room.
   a. Set up chairs and tables.
   b. Place a Prayer Partner Request Form on each chair.
   c. Have extra pens or pencils, paper and Bibles available for those who might have forgotten them.

THE MEETING

1. **Arrival Activity—15 Minutes**
   a. Greet and encourage each member.
   b. Weigh members, record weights and listen to Scripture memory verse recitations.
   c. Collect the CRs and return the evaluated ones.
   d. Direct members to complete new Prayer Partner Request Forms and place them in the container.
   e. Open in prayer.
   f. **Optional**: View the *Nine Commitments* video segment as members are arriving and weighing in.
2. **Wellness Spotlight—15 Minutes**
   Discuss the Wellness Worksheet: Eating Habits Inventory.
   a. Invite members to share what changes they are ready to make in their eating habits.
   b. Allow others to share how they have been successful in changing eating patterns.

3. **Bible Study—30 Minutes**

    Facilitate a discussion of week three of the Bible study.

4. **At-Home Assignments**

    Instruct members to complete the following assignments before the next meeting:

    a. Complete week four of the Bible study.

    b. Read and complete the Wellness Worksheets.

        1) Preventing Osteoporosis (pp. 149-151, MG)

        2) Starting a Walking Program (pp. 91-92, MG)

        3) How Physically Active Are You? (pp. 82-84, MG)

    c. Memorize this week's Scripture memory verse.

    d. Encourage one other group member.

    e. Complete the CR.

5. **Prayer Time—10 Minutes**

    a. Ask for prayer requests and praises. Remind members to record requests on the Group Prayer Requests page at the end of week four in the Bible study.

    b. Have each member select a Prayer Partner Request Form from the container.

    c. Close in prayer.

AFTER THE MEETING

1. Evaluate members' CRs.
2. Calculate weight loss for each member and determine the group total for the week.
3. Contact absentees by phone or note, encouraging them to attend next week and informing them of the At-Home Assignments for the week.

GROUP MEETING WEEK SIX

LEARNING ACTIVITIES	AT-HOME ASSIGNMENTS
Preventing Osteoporosis *Starting a Walking Program* *Discussion of week four of the Bible study*	*SL: Changing Recipes* *Calculating Exchanges for a Recipe* *EM: Understanding Weight Gain and Obesity—* *Part II*

BEFORE THE MEETING

1. Review the Wellness Worksheets and highlight or make a list of the points you plan to emphasize.

   a. Preventing Osteoporosis (pp. 149-151, MG)

   b. Starting a Walking Program (pp. 91-92, MG)

2. Select one of the following options for this week's Wellness Spotlight:

   a. Research the importance of calcium. Collect foods and labels containing calcium to bring to class.

   b. Invite a personal trainer or fitness expert to talk about developing a walking program.

   c. Recruit someone to speak on the value of walking for exercise or to give a personal testimony.

3. Complete week four of the Bible study.
   Use the leader's guide at the back of the Bible study to prepare a discussion.

4. Memorize the Scripture memory verse.

5. Arrive early to set up the room.

   a. Set up chairs and tables.

   b. Place a Prayer Partner Request Form on each chair.

   c. Have extra pens or pencils, paper and Bibles available for those who might have forgotten them.

THE MEETING

1. **Arrival Activity—15 Minutes**

   a. Greet and encourage each member.

   b. Weigh members, record weights and listen to Scripture memory verse recitations.

   c. Collect the CRs and return the evaluated ones.

   d. Direct members to complete new Prayer Partner Request Forms and place them in the container.

   e. Open in prayer.

   f. **Optional**: View the *Nine Commitments* video segment as members are arriving and weighing in.

2. **Wellness Spotlight—15 Minutes**

   a. Discuss the Wellness Worksheets.

      1) Preventing Osteoporosis.

      2) Starting a Walking Program.

   b. Introduce the option you chose for this portion of the meeting. **Note:** Depending on which option you chose, you may need to adjust the time for this segment.

3. **Bible Study—30 Minutes**

   Facilitate a discussion of week four of the Bible study.

4. **At-Home Assignments**

   Instruct members to complete the following assignments before the next meeting:

   a. Complete week five of the Bible study.

   b. Read and complete the Wellness Worksheets.

      1) Changing Recipes (pp. 141-143, *MG*).

      2) Calculating Exchanges for a Recipe (pp. 147-148, *MG*).

      3) Understanding Weight Gain and Obesity—Part III (pp. 118-120, *MG*).

   c. Memorize this week's Scripture memory verse.

   d. Encourage one other group member.

   e. Complete the CR.

5. **Prayer Time—15 Minutes**

   a. Ask for prayer requests and praises. Remind members to record requests on the Group Prayer Requests page at the end of week five in the Bible study.

   b. Have each member select a Prayer Partner Request Form from the container.

   c. Close in prayer.

AFTER THE MEETING

1. Evaluate members' CRs.
2. Calculate weight loss for each member and determine the group total for the week.
3. Contact absentees by phone or note, encouraging them to attend next week and informing them of the At-Home Assignments for the week.

GROUP MEETING WEEK SEVEN

LEARNING ACTIVITIES	AT-HOME ASSIGNMENTS
Changing Recipes *Calculating Exchanges for a Recipe* *Discussion of week five of the Bible study*	*SL: The Anytime, Anywhere Restaurant Guide* *EM: Testing Your Health-Related Fitness* *Monitoring Your Exercise Intensity*

BEFORE THE MEETING

1. Review the Wellness Worksheets and highlight or make a list of the points you plan to emphasize.
   a. Changing Recipes (pp. 141-143, MG)
   b. Calculating Exchanges for a Recipe (pp. 147-148, MG)
2. Make copies, one for each member, of the Mexican Pizza Recipe conversion chart (p. 147, MG). **Optional**: Make an overhead transparency of the conversion chart for ease in discussion.
3. Complete week five of the Bible study.
   Use the leader's guide at the back of the Bible study to prepare a discussion.
4. Memorize the Scripture memory verse
5. Arrive early to set up the room.
   a. Set up chairs and tables. If you plan to use an overhead transparency, set up a projector and screen.
   b. Place a Prayer Partner Request Form on each chair.
   c. Have extra pens or pencils, paper and Bibles available for those who might have forgotten them.

THE MEETING

1. **Arrival Activity—15 Minutes**
   a. Greet and encourage each member.
   b. Weigh members, record weights and listen to Scripture memory verse recitations.
   c. Collect the CRs and return the evaluated ones.
   d. Direct members to complete new Prayer Partner Request Forms and place them in the container.
   e. Open in prayer.
   f. **Optional**: View the *Nine Commitments* video segment as members are arriving and weighing in.

2. **Wellness Spotlight—15 Minutes**

   Discuss the Wellness Worksheets.

   a. Changing Recipes

      1) Ask members what suggestions would benefit their efforts to cook healthier without sacrificing good taste.

      2) Invite group members to share tips not listed on the worksheet.

   b. Calculating Exchanges for a Recipe

      1) Hand out copies of the Mexican Pizza Recipe conversion chart (or use the overhead transparency). Remind members that they can make copies of the one in the *Member's Guide* for use at home.

      2) Using the information found in the Calculating Exchange for a Recipe worksheet, teach members how to exchange the recipe. Have members refer to the food lists in the Live-It Food Plan in their member's guide to determine how each ingredient is exchanged.

3. **Bible Study—30 minutes**

   Facilitate a discussion of week five of the Bible study.

4. **At-Home Assignments**

   Instruct members to complete the following assignments before the next meeting:

   a. Complete week six of the Bible study.

   b. Read and complete the Wellness Worksheets.

      1) The Anytime, Anywhere Restaurant Guide (pp. 138-140, MG)

      2) Testing Your Health-Related Fitness (pp. 85-90, MG)

      3) Monitoring Your Exercise Intensity (pp. 102-104, MG)

   c. Complete week four of the Bible study.

   d. Memorize this week's Scripture memory verse.

   e. Encourage one other group member.

   f. Complete the CR.

5. **Prayer Time—15 Minutes**

   a. Ask for prayer requests and praises. Remind members to record requests on the Group Prayer Requests page at the end of week six in the Bible study.

   b. Have each member select a Prayer Partner Request Form from the container.

   c. Close in prayer.

After the Meeting

1. Evaluate members' CRs.
2. Calculate weight loss for each member and determine the group total for the week.
3. Contact absentees by phone or note, encouraging them to attend next week and informing them of the At-Home Assignments for the week.

GROUP MEETING WEEK EIGHT

LEARNING ACTIVITIES	AT-HOME ASSIGNMENTS
The Anytime, Anywhere Restaurant Guide	*SL: Sugar—Sweetness by Any Other Name*
Discussion of week six of the Bible study	*EM: Fitting in Strength Training*
	A Wellness Worksheet from the Bible study

BEFORE THE MEETING

1. Review the Wellness Worksheets: The Anytime, Anywhere Restaurant Guide (pp. 138-140, MG) and highlight or make a list of the points you plan to emphasize.

2. Prepare for a group activity using restaurant menus.

   a. Gather menus from area restaurants for a group activity.

   b. Place each menu in its own large envelope with an index card on which you have written the following directions:

   > Your mission—should you choose to accept it—is to order a meal from this menu that has three meat exchanges, two bread exchanges, one vegetable exchange and one fat exchange.

   c. On the outside of each envelope write "Mission: Impossible."

3. Determine which Wellness Worksheet from the Bible study to use for the Extra Mile assignment.

4. Complete week six of the Bible study.
   Use the leader's guide at the back of the Bible study to prepare a discussion.

5. Memorize the Scripture memory verse.

6. Arrive early to set up the room.

   a. Set up chairs and tables.

   b. Place a Prayer Partner Request Form on each chair.

   c. Have extra pens or pencils, paper and Bibles available for those who might have forgotten them.

THE MEETING

1. **Arrival Activity—15 Minutes**

   a. Greet and encourage each member.

   b. Weigh members, record weights and listen to Scripture memory verse recitations.

   c. Collect the CRs and return the evaluated ones.

   d. Direct members to complete new Prayer Partner Request Forms and place them in the container.

   e. Open in prayer.

   f. **Optional**: View the *Nine Commitments* video segment as members are arriving and weighing in.

2. **Wellness Spotlight—15 Minutes**

   a. Briefly summarize the main points of the Wellness Worksheet: The Anytime, Anywhere Restaurant Guide.

   b. Introduce the Mission: Impossible activity.

      1) Instruct members to form small groups of three or four.

      2) Give each group one envelope containing restaurant menu and their mission.

      3) Allow 10 minutes for groups to complete the activity.

      4) Have each group share their choices and how they exchanged each item ordered.

3. **Bible Study—30 Minutes**

   Facilitate a discussion of week six of the Bible study.

4. **At-Home Assignments**

   Instruct members to complete the following assignments before the next meeting:

   a. Complete week seven of the Bible Study.

   b. Read and complete the Wellness Worksheets.

      1) Sugar—Sweetness by Any Other Name (pp. 135-137, MG)

      2) Fitting in Strength Training (pp. 105-107, MG)

      3) The assigned leader's choice Wellness Worksheet from the Bible study

   c. Memorize the Scripture verse.

   d. Encourage one other group member.

   e. Complete the CR.

 **Note:** Ask for a volunteer to bring a First Place dessert for next week. Provide a copy of either of the two recipes at the end of this section, or visit First Place's web site at www.firstplace.org for more ideas.

---

5. **Prayer Time—15 Minutes**
    a. Ask for prayer requests and praises. Remind members to record requests on the Group Prayer Requests page at the end of week seven in the Bible study.
    b. Have each member select a Prayer Partner Request Form from the container.
    c. Close in prayer.

AFTER THE MEETING

1. Evaluate members' CRs.
2. Calculate weight loss for each member and determine the group total for the week.
3. Contact absentees by phone or note, encouraging them to attend next week and informing them of the At-Home Assignments for the week.

Blue Ribbon Frozen Snickers

12 oz. frozen vanilla yogurt
    or ice cream (fat-free, sugar-free)

1 small box sugar-free chocolate
    pudding, dry

3 graham cracker squares

1 cup Cool Whip Lite

3 tbsp. chunky peanut butter

Crush graham crackers into fine crumbs and place in an 8x8-inch baking dish. Mix all other ingredients together. Carefully pour into dish, so as not to disturb crumbs. Freeze until firm. Remove from freezer 10 minutes before serving. Cut into 8 equal portions.

Exchange Value: ½ meat exchange + 1 bread exchange + ½ fat exchange

Source

Chocolate Éclair Dessert

24 low-fat graham crackers
    (approximately 1 box)

1 small box sugar-free instant
    chocolate pudding

4 ½ cups skim milk

12 oz. Cool Whip Lite, thawed

2 small boxes sugar-free instant
    vanilla pudding

Place 8 graham crackers in bottom of 13x9-inch pan. Mix vanilla puddings and 3 cups milk well; let sit 2 minutes. Gently fold in Cool Whip. Pour half on graham crackers. Top with another 8 crackers. Pour remaining mixture; top with remaining crackers. Mix the chocolate pudding with 1 ½ cups milk; let sit 2 minutes. Spread over graham crackers. Let sit 6 hours or overnight in a refrigerator to soften crackers. Strawberries may be served on top as a garnish.

Exchange Value: 1 bread exchange + ¼ milk exchange + ½ fat exchange

Source

GROUP MEETING WEEK NINE

LEARNING ACTIVITIES	AT-HOME ASSIGNMENTS
Sugar—Sweetness by Any Other Name *Discussion of week seven of the Bible study*	*SL: The Truth About Fats* *EM: Running Your Way to Health and Fitness* *A Wellness Worksheet from the Bible study*

BEFORE THE MEETING

1. Review the Wellness Worksheet: Sugar—Sweetness by Any Other Name (pp. 135-137, MG) and highlight or make a list of points you plan to emphasize.
   a. Review "Sweet Sally." Plan to use sugar packets or a cup of sugar for demonstration of sugar as the story is read at the meeting. Collect any props you plan to use such as a plate, a spoon, etc.
   b. Collect different types of artificial sweeteners to show during the meeting.
2. Determine which Wellness Worksheet from the Bible study to use for the Extra Mile assignment.
3. Call and remind the member who volunteered to make the dessert. Bring napkins, plates/bowls and utensils for the dessert.
4. Complete week seven of the Bible study.
   Use the leader's guide at the back of the Bible study to prepare a discussion.
5. Memorize the Scripture memory verse.
6. Arrive early to set up the room.
   a. Set up chairs and tables.
   b. Place a Prayer Partner Request Form on each chair.
   c. Have extra pens or pencils, paper and Bibles available for those who might have fo gotten them.

THE MEETING

1. **Arrival Activity—15 Minutes**
   a. Greet and encourage each member.
   b. Weigh members, record weights and listen to Scripture memory verse recitations.
   c. Collect the CRs and return the evaluated ones.
   d. Direct members to complete new Prayer Partner Request Forms and place them in the container.
   e. Open in prayer.
   f. **Optional**: View the *Nine Commitments* video segment as members are arriving and weighing in.

2. **Wellness Spotlight—15 Minutes**

   Discuss the Wellness Worksheet: Sugar—Sweetness by Any Other Name:

   a. Point out the different artificial sweeteners you have brought. Make it very clear that each First Place member will have to make a personal choice about the use of sweeteners. These have been approved because scientific evidence does not support various concerns reported by some individuals.

   b. Mention that substituting artificial sweeteners for sugar in recipes is a little tricky, but do-able. The consistency of the recipe is affected and using applesauce along with the artificial sweetener often works well in place of the sugar in a recipe.

   c. Give toll-free numbers found on the packages to call for free recipes and cooking tips for each type of artificial sweetener.

   d. Read "Sweet Sally" on the following page. Ask some one to assist you in demonstrating as you place the appropriate number of sugar packets or teaspoons of sugar on a plate each time an amount of sugar is mentioned.

   e. Emphasize that choosing to use sugar in moderation is completely acceptable in the First Place program. Health officials suggest no more than 10 percent of total calories should be from sweets, and sweets should not replace any nutritional food exchanges such as counting sugar as a fruit.

3. **Bible Study—30 Minutes**

   Facilitate a discussion of week seven of the Bible study.

4. **At-Home Assignments**

   Instruct members to complete the following assignments before the next meeting:

   a. Complete week eight of the Bible study.

   b. Read and complete the Wellness Worksheets.

      1) The Truth About Fats (pp. 152-154, MG)

      2) Running Your Way to Health and Fitness (pp. 93-95, MG)

      3) The assigned leader's choice Wellness Worksheet from the Bible study

   c. Memorize this week's Scripture memory verse.

   d. Encourage one other group member.

   e. Complete the CR.

5. **Prayer Time—15 Minutes**

   a. Ask for prayer requests and praises. Remind members to record requests on the Group Prayer Requests page at the end of week eight in the Bible study.

   b. Have each member select a Prayer Partner Request Form from the container.

   c. Close in prayer.

   d. Invite members to enjoy a serving of the dessert.

AFTER THE MEETING

1. Evaluate members' CRs.
2. Calculate weight loss for each member and determine the group total for the week.
3. Contact absentees by phone or note, encouraging them to attend next week and informing them of the At-Home Assignments for the week.

SWEET SALLY

Let's look at the diet of an average lady, Sweet Sally. She likes to start her day with a nutritious breakfast. She passes up the donut she really wanted and eats a bowl of cereal. Neglecting to take a close look at the nutritional information on the box, she doesn't realize that one bowl of presweetened cereal has eight teaspoons of sugar. Add to this the seven teaspoons in her slice of white toast and jam and the four in the grapefruit juice she drinks—it's only 7:30 A.M., and she's had *nineteen* teaspoons of sugar!

Sweet Sally has a midmorning break at the office and sticks with just a couple of cups of coffee, but she just can't pass up that delicious flavored nonfat creamer—which adds another six teaspoons of sugar.

At lunch she decides to eat light and enjoys a bowl of chicken soup—included free are four teaspoons of sugar. A gelatin dessert adds another four and a glass of presweetened lemonade contributes a whopping eight!

On the way to driving the kids to soccer practice, she stops at a convenience store. Since lunch was so light, she decides she needs a snack too, but she at least sticks with fat-free cookies and a soda. No big deal—she used to drink three or four sodas a day. The small package of fat-free, creme-filled sandwich cookies added four teaspoons of sugar and the soda another ten!

She and the kids get home from practice too late to cook, so she fixes a frozen beef dinner, complete with fries and catsup—one of her family's favorites. Since she has had hardly any fat today she eats the same. That's another five teaspoons of sugar, and a small dish of sherbet adds eight more. At least she didn't eat the cherry pie a la mode that her husband chose! One piece would have added an unbelievable twenty teaspoons of sugar.

Sweet Sally's total for the day? Sixty-six teaspoons of sugar in a diet that is sadly representative of many Americans today.

GROUP MEETING WEEK TEN

LEARNING ACTIVITIES	AT-HOME ASSIGNMENTS
The Truth About Fats *Assigned Leader's Choice Wellness Worksheet* *Discussion of week eight Bible study*	*SL: Choosing High Fiber Foods* *Meatless Meals* *EM: Bicycling Your Way to Health and Fitness*

BEFORE THE MEETING

1. Review the Wellness Worksheets and highlight or make a list of the points you plan to emphasize.
   a. The Truth About Fats (pp. 152-154, MG)
   b. The assigned leader's choice Wellness Worksheet from the Bible Study
2. Read over the "A Day Full of Fat" and make plans to illustrate the story. You will need to bring the following items to the meeting:
   a. Liquid cooking oil
   b. Two clear glass bowls
   c. A teaspoon
   d. The story "A Day Full of Fat" (p. 00) for a member to read while you dip out the spoonfuls of fat
2. Complete week eight of the Bible study.
   Use the leader's guide at the back of the Bible study to prepare a discussion.
3. Memorize the Scripture memory verse
5. Arrive early to set up the room.
   a. Set up chairs and tables.
   b. Place a Prayer Partner Request Form on each chair.
   c. Have extra pens or pencils, paper and Bibles available for those who might have forgotten them.
   d. Set up table for the "A Day Full of Fat" demonstration. Pour oil into one of the bowls and place both bowls on the table with the teaspoon.

THE MEETING

1. **Arrival Activity—15 Minutes**
   a. Greet and encourage each member.
   b. Weigh members, record weights and listen to Scripture memory verse recitations.

c. Collect the CRs and return the evaluated ones.

d. Direct members to complete new Prayer Partner Request Forms and place them in the container.

e. Open in prayer.

f. **Optional:** View the *Nine Commitments* video segment as members are arriving and weighing in.

2. **Wellness Spotlight—15 Minutes**

Discuss the Wellness Worksheets.

a. The Truth About Fats

Enlist a member to read "A Day Full of Fat" as you illustrate by dipping out teaspoons of oil from one bowl to another.

b. The assigned leader's choice Wellness Worksheet

3. **Bible Study—30 Minutes**

Facilitate a discussion of week eight of the Bible study.

4. **At-Home Assignments**

Instruct members to complete the following assignments before the next meeting:

a. Complete week nine of the Bible Study.

b. Read and complete the Wellness Worksheets.

1) Choosing High Fiber Foods (pp. 155-157, MG)

2) Meatless Meals (pp. 144-146, MG)

3) Bicycling Your Way to Health and Fitness (pp. 96-98, MG)

c. Memorize this week's Scripture memory verse.

d. Encourage one other group member.

e. Complete the CR.

5. **Prayer Time—15 Minutes**

a. Ask for prayer requests and praises. Remind members to record requests on the Group Prayer Requests page at the end of week nine in the Bible study.

b. Have each member select a Prayer Partner Request Form from the container.

c. Close in prayer.

AFTER THE MEETING

1. Evaluate members' CRs.

2. Calculate weight loss for each member and determine the group total for the week.

3. Contact absentees by phone or note, encouraging them to attend next week and informing them of the At-Home Assignments for the week.

A DAY FULL OF FAT

Let's take a look at an average day in the life of Saturated Sam. He starts his day off at home with what he believes is an all-American breakfast of a three-egg, ham and cheese omelet. A grand total of seven teaspoons of fat, including the tablespoon of oil it was cooked in. Two slices of buttered toast add three more, plus one in his glass of milk.

A mid-morning donut adds another seven teaspoons, but Sam is feeling just a little righteous about his choice. *Now what other man would only choose one donut?* he thinks to himself.

Lunch is on the road. Sam stops by his favorite fast food restaurant and orders his favorite meal deal. He chuckles to himself about what a bargain it is to supersize. The hamburger adds six teaspoons of fat and the super-sized French fries another six. What a bargain for less than five dollars! The candy-filled ice cream treat adds another five. This popular lunch for millions of Americans each day has a total of seventeen teaspoons of fat—and more that half of that fat was saturated.

Sam skips an afternoon snack, still feeling rather full. He gets home that night to one of his favorite meals: sirloin steak, baked potato and broccoli with cheese sauce, salad and two rolls. Let's add five teaspoons of fat for the six-ounce steak, eight more teaspoons for his choice of potato toppings: butter, sour cream, bacon bits and cheese. The cheese-sauce topping—or maybe we should say "drowning"—on his broccoli adds another two. We need to add six teaspoons for the two tablespoons of dressing on that delicious salad. Add two more for the fat in the rolls, and another four for the two teaspoons of butter he added to each roll. Saturated Sam picks up his favorite fried pie at the store which adds another four teaspoons of fat to his evening meal.

After watching a few hours of TV, vigorously working that remote control from his recliner, Sam begins to feel just a little hungry. He remembers that six-ounce steak was a bit on the small side, so he figures he deserves his regular bowl of ice cream, adding another five teaspoons of fat, before heading off to bed.

Total for the day? Seventy-one teaspoons of fat—more than half were saturated fats—in this not so unusual day of an American man. It is not so surprising that Americans lead the world in heart disease and other health-related illnesses resulting from an everyday diet of too much fat.

GROUP MEETING WEEK ELEVEN

LEARNING ACTIVITIES	AT-HOME ASSIGNMENTS
Choosing High-Fiber Foods *Meatless Meals* *Discussion of week nine of the Bible study*	*SL: Off to a Good Start* *Sharing Your Faith* *EM: Water Exercise for Health and Fitness*

BEFORE THE MEETING

1. Review the Wellness Worksheets and highlight or make a list of the points you plan to emphasize.
    a. Choosing High-Fiber Foods (pp. 155-157, MG)
        1) Prepare high-fiber muffins and print out the recipe to share during the meeting.
        2) Gather examples of foods that are both low and high in fiber.
    b. Meatless Meals (pp. 144-146, MG)
2. Complete week nine of the Bible study.
    Use the leader's guide at the back of the Bible study to prepare a discussion.
3. Memorize the Scripture memory verse.
4. Arrive early to set up the room.
    a. Set up chairs and tables.
    b. Place a Prayer Partner Request Form on each chair.
    c. Have extra pens or pencils, paper and Bibles available for those who might have forgotten them.
    d. Bring napkins for serving the muffins.

The Meeting

1. **Arrival Activity—15 Minutes**
    a. Greet and encourage each member.
    b. Weigh members, record weights and listen to Scripture memory verse recitations
    c. Collect the CRs and return the evaluated ones.
    d. Direct members to complete new Prayer Partner Request Forms and place them in the container.
    e. Open in prayer.
    f. **Optional:** View the *Nine Commitments* video segment as members are arriving and weighing in.
2. **Wellness Spotlight—15 Minutes**
    Discuss the Wellness Worksheets.

    a. Choosing High-Fiber Foods

        1) Review the difference between soluble fiber and insoluble fiber.

        2) Have members brainstorm ways they can increase fiber in their diets.

        3) Show examples of high- and low-fiber foods.

        4) Ask members to begin filling out their CRs during the meeting and direct them to write "Eat more fiber!" on the bottom of the cover page. (This will be their goal for the week.)

    b. Meatless Meals

3. **Bible Study—30 Minutes**

Facilitate a discussion of week nine of the Bible study.

4. **At-Home Assignments**

Instruct members to complete the following assignments before the next meeting:

    a. Complete week 10 of the Bible study.

    b. Read and complete the Wellness Worksheets.

        1) Sharing Your Faith (pp. 26-28, MG)

        2) Off to a Good Start (pp. 158-160, MG)

        3) Water Exercise for Fitness and Health (pp. 99-101, MG)

    c. Memorize this week's Scripture memory verse.

    d. Encourage one other group member.

    e. Complete the CR.

5. **Prayer Time—15 Minutes**

    a. Ask for prayer requests and praises. Remind members to record requests on the Group Prayer Requests page at the end of week 10 in the Bible study.

    b. Have each member select a Prayer Partner Request Form from the container.

    c. Close in prayer.

    d. Invite members to enjoy a muffin.

AFTER THE MEETING

1. Evaluate members' CRs.
2. Calculate weight loss for each member and determine the group total for the week.
3. Contact absentees by phone or note, encouraging them to attend next week and informing them of the At-Home Assignments for the week.

Oatmeal Banana Muffins

3 cups whole-wheat flour
¾ cup rolled oats
1 tbsp. baking powder
½ tsp. ground cinnamon
¼ tsp. ground nutmeg
1 tbsp. sugar

1 egg
2 tbsp. vegetable oil
1 ½ cups nonfat milk
1 small banana, cubed
¼ cup sunflower seeds, toasted

Combine the flour, oats, baking powder, cinnamon, nutmeg and sugar in a bowl. Add the remaining ingredients and blend. Spoon into oiled or paper-lined muffin tins. Bake at 375° F for 15 to 20 minutes. Yields 12 servings.

One muffin: calories = 180; carbohydrates = 29; protein = 5; fat = 5; sodium = 91; potassium = 221; cholesterol = 23.

Exchange Value: 1 bread exchange + 1 fruit exchange + 1 fat exchange

Source
Betty Wedman, M.S., R.D., *Holiday Cookbook*, American Diabetes Association
© 2001 Gospel Light. Permission to photocopy granted. *First Place Leader's Guide*

GROUP MEETING WEEK TWELVE

LEARNING ACTIVITIES	AT-HOME ASSIGNMENTS
Off to a Good Start *Sharing Your Faith* *Discussion of week ten of the Bible study*	*SL: Write a personal testimony using Sharing Your Faith*

BEFORE THE MEETING

1. Review the Wellness Worksheets and highlight or make a list of the points you plan to emphasize.
   a. Off to a Good Start (pp. 158-160, MG)
   b. Sharing Your Faith (pp. 26-28, MG)
      Prepare your personal testimony to share with the group and/or select a member who is willing to share a brief testimony with the group.
2. Prepare a sign-up sheet for members to bring food or other items (e.g., paper goods, decorations, ice, etc.) for the Victory Celebration.
3. Complete week 10 of the Bible study.
   Use the leader's guide at the back of the Bible study to prepare a discussion.
4. Memorize the Scripture memory verse.
5. Arrive early to set up the room.
   a. Set up chairs and tables.
   b. Place a Prayer Partner Request Form on each chair.
   c. Have extra pens or pencils, paper and Bibles available for those who might have forgotten them.

THE MEETING

1. **Arrival Activity—15 Minutes**
   a. Greet and encourage each member.
   b. Weigh members, record weights and listen to Scripture memory verse recitations.
   c. Collect the CRs and return the evaluated ones.
   d. Direct members to complete new Prayer Partner Request Forms and place them in the container.
   e. Open in prayer.
   f. **Optional**: View the *Nine Commitments* video segment as members are arriving and weighing in.

2. **Wellness Spotlight—15 Minutes**

   Discuss the Wellness Worksheets.

   a. Off to a Good Start

      1) Share examples of healthy breakfast choices.

      2) Ask members to share breakfast ideas.

      3) Use the example of a campfire: You must continually feed the fire to keep it burning. You can't let it burn down and then put a big log on the fire because that would put the fire out. So it is with our bodies: If we don't eat for a while and then load up on food in one meal, our bodies can't burn the calories properly—in effect, putting the fire (our energy) out.

   b. Sharing Your Faith: Share your testimony and/or invite a volunteer to share.

3. **Bible Study—30 Minutes**

   Facilitate a discussion of week 10 of the Bible Study.

4. **At-Home Assignments**

   Instruct members to complete the following assignments before the next meeting:

   a. Write a personal testimony on the Sharing Your Faith Wellness Worksheet.

   b. Review the 10 Scripture memory verses learned over the entire session.

   c. Prepare their personal testimonies to share at Group Celebration.

   d. Sign up to bring food or other item (i.e., paper goods, decorations, ice, etc.) for the Victory Celebration.

   e. Encourage one other group member.

   f. Complete the CR.

5. **Prayer Time—15 Minutes**

   a. Ask for prayer requests and praises. Remind members to record requests on the Group Prayer Requests page at the end of week 10 in the Bible study.

   b. Have each member select a Prayer Partner Request Form from the container.

   c. Close in prayer.

AFTER THE MEETING

1. Evaluate members' CRs.
2. Calculate weight loss for each member and determine the group total for the week.
3. Contact absentees by phone or note, encouraging them to attend next week and informing them of the At-Home Assignments for the week.

GROUP MEETING WEEK THIRTEEN

> ## LEARNING ACTIVITIES
>
> *Sharing testimonies of Christ's work in members' lives*
> *Celebrate victories*
> *Recognize achievements of individual members*

BEFORE THE MEETING

1. Call and remind members of food or other items they signed up to bring for the Victory Celebration. During the phone call, ask for volunteers to share all 10 of the Scripture Memory verses.
2. Make arrangements for the meeting room set-up for the Victory Celebration.
3. Secure decorations, paper products, tablecloths, etc.
4. Coordinate any music or other entertainment that you have planned.
5. Arrive early and prepare room. It is suggested that you recruit extra help from group members.

THE MEETING

1. **Arrival Activity—15 Minutes**
   a. Greet and encourage each member.
   b. Weigh members, record weights and listen to Scripture memory verse recitations.
   c. Collect the CRs and return the evaluated ones.
   d. Direct members to complete new Prayer Partner Request Forms and place them in the container.
   e. Open in prayer.
2. **The Celebration**
   a. Enjoy the meal.
   b. Have entertainers perform.
   c. Invite volunteers to share salvation testimonies as prepared as part of the Sharing Your Faith worksheets.
   d. Invite others to share their First Place testimonies.
   e. Present achievement awards.
   f. Conclude with encouraging words and invite members to return for the next session, announcing the time and place.
   g. Close in group prayer.

After the Meeting

1. Evaluate members' CRs.
2. Calculate weight loss for each member and determine the group total for the week.
3. Begin preparation for the next session of First Place!

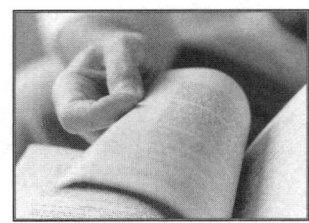

Reproducible Leadership Forms and Samples

LAST CHANCE TO BE A LOSER

Lose weight and feel great this summer!

**The losers are the winners with First Place,
a Christ-centered health and weight-loss program.**

*Orientation Meeting, Tuesday, June 8, 6:00 p.m.
in the Arts and Crafts room at First Church*

Orientation is required for new members.

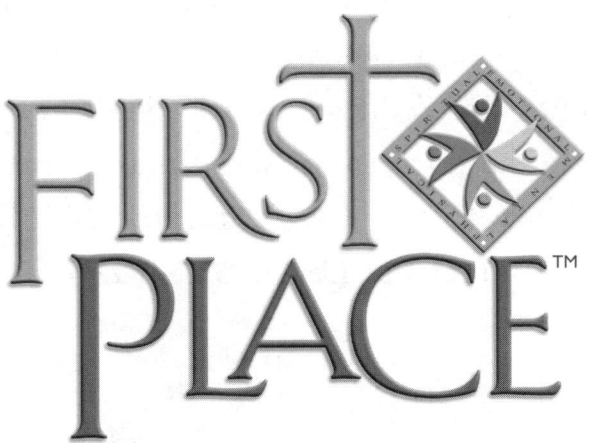

Summer Session Schedule:
Group Session begins June 8 and end August 17.
Meetings offered Tuesdays at noon and in the evening.

For more information call the church office 555-5555.

It's Coming! Don't Miss It!

Do you want to improve your relationships with others? Do you desire to be physically fit? Would you like to know God in a more intimate way? Well, the answer to all of these desires is coming!

First Place, a Christ-centered health program, is one of the premier total-wellness programs, and you have the awesome opportunity to be a part of this exciting ministry. To find out how to achieve emotional, physical, mental and spiritual health, register today for the First Place group at the College of Biblical Studies.

This semester there will be two 13-week sessions offered beginning the week of January 29 on Mondays from 7:00 P.M. to 8:30 P.M. or Wednesdays from 9:30 A.M. to 11:00 A.M. To join, attend an informational orientation meeting on Monday, January 15 at 7:30 P.M. in room 205. **For more information, contact Pat Lewis, 555-1234, ext. 10.**

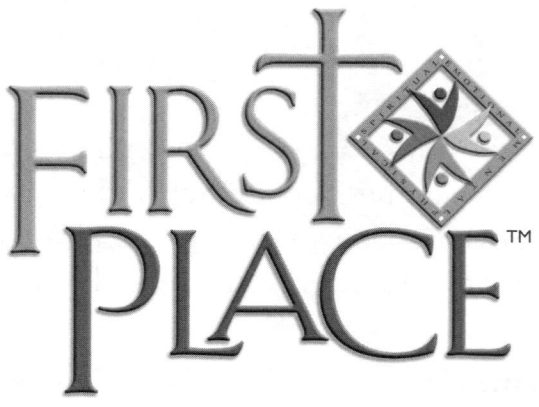

JOIN FIRST PLACE: A CHRIST-CENTERED HEALTH PROGRAM

HOUSTON'S FIRST BAPTIST CHURCH

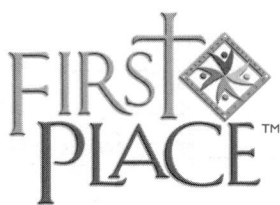

Again this fall, First Place offers you 13 weeks of instruction and support. To join, you must attend one of the orientation meetings:

Tuesday, August 13, at 7 P.M. in the Chapel
Sunday, August 25, at 5 P.M. in the Chapel

The First Place program combines Bible study and Scripture reading with a sensible eating plan to help all participants focus on giving Christ first place in every area of their lives. The ultimate goal is for each person to experience more abundant life, as Christ becomes Lord of the spiritual, mental, emotional and physical lives of His children.

The cost for first-time members will be $_____. This includes: registration, the *Member's Guide*, four audiocassettes, *Choosing to Change*, *First Place Journal*, *Scripture Memory Verse Book*, Commitment Records and the first Bible study.

Continuing members in the First Place program must turn in preregistration forms with a $_____ registration fee by August 20th to assure your spot in the fall session at the following locations:

All meetings will start the week of September 3rd.
Groups will be offered at the following times:

Sundays, 5:15-6:30 P.M.—Women's and coed classes available (nursery provided)
Tuesdays, 12:00 noon-1:15 P.M.—Women (nursery provided for a $10.00 fee)
Tuesdays, 7:00-8:15 P.M.—Women's and coed classes available (nursery provided)
Wednesdays, 4:45-6:00 P.M.—Coed (nursery provided)
Thursdays, 6:15-7:30 A.M.—Coed (no nursery provided)
Saturdays, 10:00-11:15 A.M.—Women (no nursery provided)

For further information, please call the church office.

FIRST PLACE REGISTRATION FORM

Meeting Day _____ ☐ New Member ☐ Male

Meeting Time _____ ☐ Alumnus ☐ Female

Leader _____

Name _____

Address _____

City _____ State _____ Zip_____

Phone Numbers (H) _____ (W) _____

Fax _____ E-mail Address _____

May we call you at work? _____

Church Member? _____ Where? _____

Would you like to receive more information about this church? _____

If provided, would you need child care? _____

Number of children and ages _____

Friends you wish to be in a group with _____

_____

Please carefully read the following statement:

    I have attended the First Place Orientation and desire to put Christ first in my life. I will do my best to follow the First Place commitments and prayerfully support other members and my leader.

    I understand that the information I will receive in the First Place program is intended to be solely informational and educational. I realize that First Place encourages participants to consult with their physicians before starting this program.

    If for any unforeseen reason I have to withdraw from the First Place program, I agree to notify my leader and discuss the matter with prayerful consideration.

Signed _____ Date _____

DO NOT WRITE BELOW THIS LINE

Paid: ☐ Yes ☐ No

Amount $ _____ Check # _____ or ☐ Cash

Class assignment: Day _____ Time_____

Leader _____

Materials Received: ☐ Yes ☐ No

Sample Letter to Alumni

(**Note**: Enclose the Preregistration for Alumni form with the letter.)

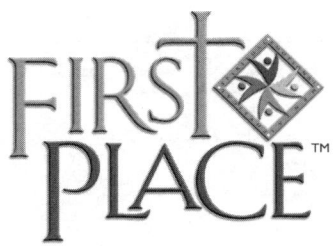

December 15, 2001

Mary Smith
231 Elmwood Ave.
Houston, Texas 77000

Dear Mary,

We would like to invite you to enroll in the winter session of First Place at Houston's First Baptist Church. This 13-week session is scheduled to begin the week of January 22 and conclude April 16, 2001. Classes will be offered Tuesdays at noon, Tuesdays at 7:00 P.M. and Wednesdays at 4:45 P.M.

The orientation meeting will be on January 7, 2001 at 4:00 P.M. in the Harbor Room. Since you are an alumnus, it is not necessary for you to attend the orientation. However, if you would like to review the commitments or bring a friend new to First Place, you are welcome to attend.

The alumni fee for this session is _____. Please complete and return the enclosed preregistration form with your check by January 15, 2001.

Sincerely,

Kay Smith

PREREGISTRATION FOR ALUMNI

Name _____ ☐ Male ☐ Female

Address _____

City _____ State _____ Zip _____

Phone Numbers (H) _____ (W) _____

Fax _____ E-mail Address _____

May we call you at work? _____

Church Member? _____ Where? _____

Would you like to receive more information about this church? _____

If provided, would you need child care? _____

Number of children and ages _____

Friends you wish to be in a group with _____

_____

Meeting Day _____ Meeting Time _____

Leader _____

Please carefully read the following statement:

I understand the commitments of the First Place program and have participated in at least one session. I have prayerfully considered my desire to continue in First Place and believe God truly is leading me to recommit myself to the Nine Commitments of the program.

I understand that the information I will receive in the First Place program is intended to be solely informational and educational. I realize that First Place encourages participants to consult with their physicians before starting this program.

If for any unforeseen reason I have to withdraw from the First Place program, I agree to notify my leader and discuss the matter with prayerful consideration.

Signed _____ Date _____

DO NOT WRITE BELOW THIS LINE

Paid: ☐ Yes ☐ No

Amount $ _____ Check # _____ or ☐ Cash

Class assignment: Day _____ Time _____

Leader _____

Materials Received: ☐ Yes ☐ No

WEEKLY LESSON PLAN FORM

Class Meeting Plan	Week	Date
Wellness Spotlight		

Wellness Worksheets	Facilitator	Materials Needed

Lesson Sequence

Bible Study

Bible Study Title	Memory Verse	Materials Needed

Lesson Sequence

Prayer Time

Previous Requests	New Requests

Session Overview

Week #	Learning Activities	At-Home Assignments
Week 1		SL: EM:
Week 2		SL: EM:
Week 3	Discuss Week One Bible Study	SL: EM:
Week 4	Discuss Week Two Bible Study	SL: EM:
Week 5	Discuss Week Three Bible Study	SL: EM:
Week 6	Discuss Week Four Bible Study	SL: EM:
Week 7	Discuss Week Five Bible Study	SL: EM:

Week #	Learning Activities	At-Home Assignments
Week 8	Discuss Week Six Bible Study	SL: EM:
Week 9	Discuss Week Seven Bible Study	SL: EM:
Week 10	Discuss Week Eight Bible Study	SL: EM:
Week 11	Discuss Week Nine Bible Study	SL: EM:
Week 12	Discuss Week Ten Bible Study	
Week 13	Victory Celebration	

First Place Group Roster

Session _____

Leader _____

Class Day _____

Time _____

Name	Address: Street, City and Zip	Home Phone	Work Phone	E-mail/Fax

Weigh-In Chart

Leader _____

Day _____ **Time** _____

Members Names	Weight Loss Goal	Week 1	Week 2	Week 3	Week 4	Week 5	Week 6	Week 7	Week 8	Week 9	Week 10	Week 11	Week 12
Weekly Loss													
Session Loss Thus Far													
Weekly Loss													
Session Loss Thus Far													
Weekly Loss													
Session Loss Thus Far													
Weekly Loss													
Session Loss Thus Far													

WEIGH-IN CHART

Leader _____ **Day** _____ **Time** _____

Members Names	Weight Loss Goal	Week 1	Week 2	Week 3	Week 4	Week 5	Week 6	Week 7	Week 8	Week 9	Week 10	Week 11	Week 12
Weekly Loss Session Loss Thus Far													
Weekly Loss Session Loss Thus Far													
Weekly Loss Session Loss Thus Far													
Total Group Loss This Week													

Total Group Loss This Session

WEIGH-IN GUIDELINES

- Keep the Weigh-In Chart concealed in a notebook or folder. Never leave it out where someone can see it.
- Weigh members in private. If possible, place scale in a separate room or in a private area of your classroom. Please don't say member's weight aloud; discreetly write the weight on the weigh-in chart.
- Ask members to recite their memory verse as they are weighed.
- Weigh members in an accurate and swift manner. Return the weight to zero before the next member is weighed.
- Be sensitive and encouraging as members weigh. Do not show a reaction to the weight on the scale, but respond to the member.
- When a member is finished weighing, remind him or her to turn in the CR.
- The Weigh-In Chart also serves as an attendance record. Weigh late arrivals after class. An exception would be a lunchtime class where members may want to weigh before they eat.
- Occasionally a member may not want to weigh in. However, always encourage him or her to view weighing in as an opportunity for a fresh start. If a member still refuses, don't insist. Simply mark him or her present on the Weigh-In Chart.

FIRST PLACE MEMBER SURVEY

FIRST PLACE MEMBER SURVEY

Please answer the following questions to help your leader plan your First Place meetings so that your needs might be met in this session. Give this form to your leader at the first meeting.

Name _____ Birth date _____

Please list those who live in your household.

Name	Relationship	Age

What church do you attend? _____

Are you interested in receiving more information about our church? ☐ Yes   ☐ No

Occupation _____

What talent or area of expertise would you be willing to share with our class?
_____
_____

Why did you join First Place? _____
_____
_____

With notice, would you be willing to lead Bible study one week? ☐ Yes   ☐ No

Are you comfortable praying out loud? _____

If the assistant leader were absent, would you be willing to assist in weighing in members and possibly evaluating the CRs? ☐ Yes   ☐ No

Any other comments?_____
_____
_____

First Place Group Meeting Evaluation

(For Leader's Use Only)

Leader _____

Date _____ Attendance _____

Week _____ Topics _____

What were the most significant events in the meeting?

What weaknesses or problems did you see in the meeting?

What did you learn that you did not know before?

What follow-up is needed (e.g., a note of encouragement, a miss-you note or a phone call)?

PRAYER PARTNER REQUEST FORM

Name _____ Week Number _____

Home Phone (_____) _____ Work Phone (_____) _____

E-mail _____

Memory Verse _____

_____

_____

Personal Prayer Concerns

✂ -

PRAYER PARTNER REQUEST FORM

Name _____ Week Number _____

Home Phone (_____) _____ Work Phone (_____) _____

E-mail _____

Memory Verse _____

_____

_____

Personal Prayer Concerns

STEPS FOR SPIRITUAL GROWTH

PRAYER

- Prayer provides spiritual food and water for *daily* living.
- Prayer helps you to give your life back to God daily.
- Prayer allows you to confess your sins daily.

   If we confess our sins, he is faithful and just and will forgive us our sins and purify us from all unrighteousness (1 John 1:9).

THE BIBLE

- Studying the Bible keeps you grounded in the essential ingredients for *daily* living.
- The Bible assures you of your salvation.

   I write these things to you who believe in the name of the Son of God so that you may know that you have eternal life (1 John 5:13).

- The Bible teaches you about the life of Jesus (read Matthew, Mark, Luke and John).

THE CHURCH

- The church provides fellowship with other believers and a place to worship God.
- Being baptized is the first step to obedience. (Matthew 3:13-17 tells of Jesus' baptism.)
- Become a member of a Bible-teaching, Bible-believing community of believers.

   So in Christ we who are many form one body, and each member belongs to all the others (Romans 12:5).

- The church is Christ's Body on earth, formed to spread the good news.

SHARING YOUR FAITH

- Jesus commanded us to lead others to Christ.

   Then Jesus came to them and said, "All authority in heaven and on earth has been given to me. Therefore go and make disciples of all nations, baptizing them in the name of the Father and of the Son and of the Holy Spirit, and teaching them to obey everything I have commanded you. And surely I am with you always, to the very end of the age" (Matthew 28:18-20).

- Sharing your faith with others is merely telling your story—how God has changed you. The Bible promises that the Holy Spirit will help you.

Now go; I will help you speak and will teach you what to say (Exodus 4:12).

Do not worry about how you will defend yourselves or what you will say, for the Holy Spirit will teach you at that time what you should say (Luke 12:11,12).

But you will receive power when the Holy Spirit comes on you; and you will be my witnesses in Jerusalem, and in all Judea and Samaria, and to the ends of the earth (Acts 1:8).

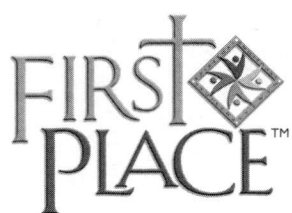

First Place Grocery List

Use this list to get you started and make copies so that you will have a list for each week.

BAKING GOODS

- ☐ ____ Baking soda
- ☐ ____ Baking powder
- ☐ ____ Cocoa
- ☐ ____ Cornstarch
- ☐ ____ Dried herbs
- ☐ ____ Nuts
- ☐ ____ Pepper
- ☐ ____ Raisins
- ☐ ____ Salt
- ☐ ____ Spices
- ☐ ____ Vanilla
- ☐ _____
- ☐ _____

BEVERAGES

- ☐ ____ Cocoa
- ☐ ____ Coffee
- ☐ ____ Fruit juice, 100%
- ☐ ____ Mineral water
- ☐ ____ Soft drinks, diet
- ☐ ____ Tea
- ☐ _____
- ☐ _____

BREADS

- ☐ ____ Bagels
- ☐ ____ Breads
- ☐ ____ Buns
- ☐ ____ English muffins
- ☐ ____ Rolls
- ☐ _____
- ☐ _____

CANNED GOODS

- ☐ ____ Applesauce
- ☐ ____ Beans
- ☐ ____ Chili
- ☐ ____ Fruit
- ☐ ____ Mushrooms
- ☐ ____ Soup
- ☐ ____ Spaghetti sauce
- ☐ ____ Stewed tomatoes
- ☐ ____ Tomato paste
- ☐ ____ Tomato sauce
- ☐ ____ Tuna/salmon
- ☐ ____ Vegetables
- ☐ _____
- ☐ _____
- ☐ _____
- ☐ _____

CONDIMENTS

- ☐ ____ All-fruit/jam/jelly
- ☐ ____ Honey
- ☐ ____ Ketchup
- ☐ ____ Low-fat
        mayonnaise
- ☐ ____ Mustard
- ☐ ____ Olive oil
- ☐ ____ Olives
- ☐ ____ Peanut butter
- ☐ ____ Pickles
- ☐ ____ Relish
- ☐ ____ Salad dressings
- ☐ ____ Salsa
- ☐ ____ Soy sauce
- ☐ ____ Syrup, diet
- ☐ ____ Vegetable oil
- ☐ ____ Vinegar

DAIRY

- ☐ ____ Butter, reduced-fat
- ☐ ____ Cream cheese
- ☐ ____ Cottage cheese
- ☐ ____ Eggs/egg sub.
- ☐ ____ Low-fat
        margarine
- ☐ ____ Low-fat sour cream
- ☐ ____ Milk, skim/1%
- ☐ ____ Other cheese
- ☐ ____ Parmesan cheese
- ☐ ____ Yogurt (90-calorie)
- ☐ _____
- ☐ _____
- ☐ _____
- ☐ _____

DRY GOODS

- [ ] _____ Beans/peas/lentils
- [ ] _____ Bread crumbs
- [ ] _____ Cereals
- [ ] _____ Cornmeal
- [ ] _____ Crackers
- [ ] _____ Flour
- [ ] _____ Oatmeal
- [ ] _____ Pancake mix
- [ ] _____ Pasta/noodles
- [ ] _____ Rice
- [ ] _____ Sugar/sugar sub.
- [ ] _____ Sugar-free pudding
- [ ] _____ Tortilla chips
- [ ] _____
- [ ] _____
- [ ] _____

FROZEN FOODS

- [ ] _____ Frozen dinners
- [ ] _____ Frozen waffles
- [ ] _____ Light whipped topping
- [ ] _____ Light yogurt/ice cream
- [ ] _____ Vegetables
- [ ] _____
- [ ] _____
- [ ] _____

FRUIT

- [ ] _____ Apples
- [ ] _____ Bananas
- [ ] _____ Berries
- [ ] _____ Grapefruit
- [ ] _____ Grapes
- [ ] _____ Lemons
- [ ] _____ Limes
- [ ] _____ Melons
- [ ] _____ Oranges
- [ ] _____ Pears
- [ ] _____
- [ ] _____
- [ ] _____

MEAT, FISH, POULTRY

- [ ] _____ Bacon, turkey
- [ ] _____ Beef, lean
- [ ] _____ Beef, lean ground
- [ ] _____ Chicken
- [ ] _____ Deli Meat
- [ ] _____ Fish
- [ ] _____ Ham, lean
- [ ] _____ Hot dogs, low fat
- [ ] _____ Pork tenderloin
- [ ] _____ Sausage, low fat
- [ ] _____ Shellfish
- [ ] _____ Turkey
- [ ] _____
- [ ] _____
- [ ] _____

VEGETABLES

- [ ] _____ Broccoli
- [ ] _____ Cabbage
- [ ] _____ Carrots
- [ ] _____ Cauliflower
- [ ] _____ Celery
- [ ] _____ Cucumbers
- [ ] _____ Garlic
- [ ] _____ Lettuce
- [ ] _____ Mushrooms
- [ ] _____ Onions
- [ ] _____ Peppers
- [ ] _____ Potatoes
- [ ] _____ Radishes
- [ ] _____ Spinach
- [ ] _____ **Tomatoes**
- [ ] _____
- [ ] _____
- [ ] _____

MISCELLANEOUS

- [ ] _____
- [ ] _____
- [ ] _____
- [ ] _____
- [ ] _____
- [ ] _____
- [ ] _____
- [ ] _____
- [ ] _____
- [ ] _____
- [ ] _____
- [ ] _____

FIRST PLACE™

REPRODUCIBLE LOGOS AND ARTWORK

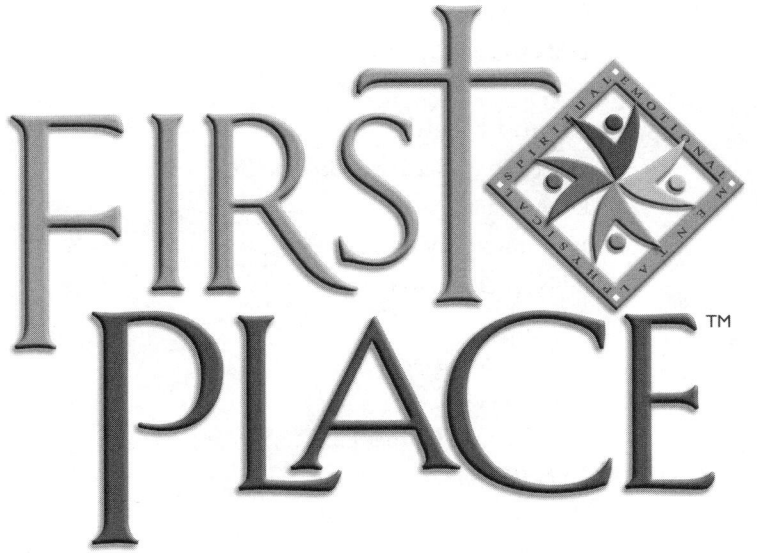

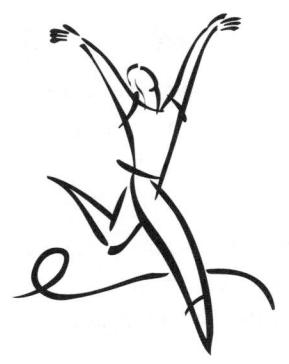

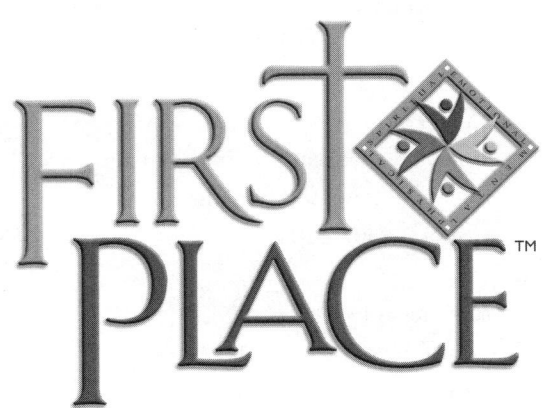

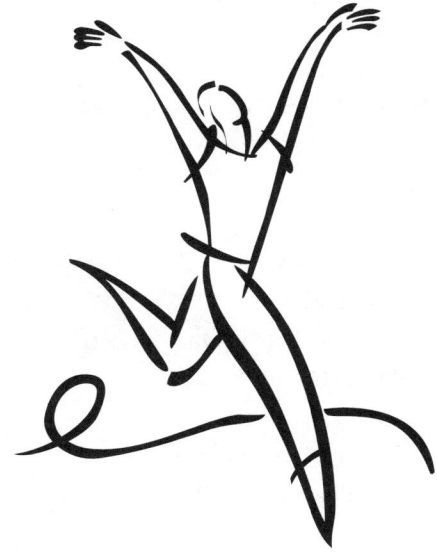

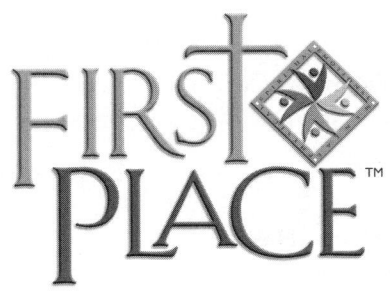

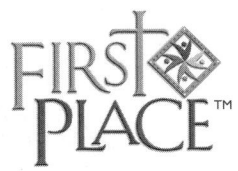

RECOMMENDED RESOURCES

Books

Emotional Health

Boundaries
Dr. Henry Cloud and Dr. Henry Townsend
Grand Rapids, MI: Zondervan Publishing House
ISBN 0-3105-8590-2

The Courage to Go On: Life After Addiction
Cynthia Rowland McClure
Grand Rapids, MI: Baker Book House
ISBN 0-8010-6263-2

The Lies We Believe
Dr. Chris Thurman
Nashville, TN: Thomas Nelson
ISBN 0-8407-3192-2

Love Hunger
Dr. Frank Minirth, Dr. Paul Meier
Grand Rapids, MI: Zondervan Publishing House
ISBN 0-3105-8590-2

Love Is a Choice
Dr. Robert Hemfelt, Dr. Frank Minirth and
Dr. Paul Meier
Nashville, TN: Thomas Nelson
ISBN 0-2407-3189-2

Winning in the Land of Giants
Dr. William Mitchell
Wheaton, IL: Tyndale House Publishers
ISBN 0-7852-8094-4

The Gift of the Blessing
Gary Smalley and John Trent, Ph.D.
Nashville, TN: Thomas Nelson
ISBN 0-8407-4849-3

Healing for Damaged Emotions
David A. Seamands
Wheaton, IL: Victor Books
ISBN 0-8820-7228-5

The Wounded Heart
Dan B. Allender
Colorado Springs, CO: NavPress
ISBN 0-8910-9289-7

Mental Health

Be the Leader You Were Meant to Be
Leroy Eims
Wheaton, IL: Victor Books
ISBN 0-8969-3168-4

Choosing to Change
Carole Lewis
Ventura, CA: Gospel Light
ISBN 0-8307-2862-7

Emotions: Can You Trust Them?
Dr. James Dobson
Ventura, CA: Regal Books
ISBN 0-8307-1662-9

First Place
Carole Lewis with W. Terry Whalin
Ventura, CA: Gospel Light
ISBN 0-8307-2863-5

See You at the Top
Zig Zigler
Westwood, NJ: H. Revell Publishers
ISBN 0-8828-9126-X

Top Performance
Zig Zigler
Gretna, LA: Pelican Publishing Company
ISBN 0-8828-9126-X

Walking in Freedom
Neil T. Anderson and Rich Miller
Ventura, CA: Regal Books
ISBN 0-8307-2394-3

What the Bible Says About Healthy Living
Rex Russell
Ventura, CA: Gospel Light
ISBN 0-8307-1858-3

Your Personality Tree
Florence Littauer
Dallas: Word Publishing
ISBN 0-8499-0571-0

Spiritual Health

Biblical Meditation for Spiritual Breakthrough
Elmer Towns
Ventura, CA: Regal Books
ISBN 0-8307-2360-9

Every Day Light
Selwyn Hughes and Thomas Kinkade
Nashville, TN: Broadman & Holman Publishers
ISBN 0-8054-0188-1

Daily Awakenings
Stephen Hill
Ventura, CA: Regal Books
ISBN 0-8307-2514-8

The Heart of Praise
Jack Hayford
Ventura, CA: Regal Books
ISBN 0-8307-1609-2

Honest to God
Bill Hybels
Grand Rapids, MI: Zondervan Publishing House
ISBN 0-3105-2180-7

A Lifestyle of Worship
David Morris
Ventura, CA: Renew
ISBN 0-8307-2199-1

Living Free in Christ
Neil T. Anderson
Ventura, CA: Regal Books
ISBN 0-8307-1639-4

Lord, Change Me
Evelyn Christianson
Wheaton, IL: Victor Books
ISBN 0-8820-7756-2

A Moment a Day
Compiled by Mary Beckwith and Kathi Mills
Ventura, CA: Regal Books
ISBN 0-8307-1288-7

My Utmost for His Highest
Oswald Chambers
Grand Rapids, MI: Discovery House Publishers
ISBN 0-9292-3957-1

One Day at a Time
Neil T. Anderson and Mike and Julia Quarles
Ventura, CA: Regal Books
ISBN 0-8307-2400-1

The One Year® Devotional
Larry Stockstill
Ventura, CA: Regal Books
ISBN 0-8307-2194-0

Praying God's Word
Beth Moore
Nashville, TN: Broadman & Holman Publishers
ISBN 0-8054-2351-6

Praying the Lord's Prayer for Spiritual Breakthrough
Elmer L. Towns
Ventura, CA: Regal Books
ISBN 0-8307-2042-1

Too Busy Not to Pray
Bill Hybels
Downers Grove, IL: InterVarsity Press
ISBN 0-8308-1256-3

Victory over the Darkness
Neil T. Anderson
Ventura, CA: Regal Books
ISBN 0-8307-1375-1
        0-8307-1669-6 (Study Guide)

Watchman Prayer
Dutch Sheets
Ventura, CA: Regal Books
ISBN 0-8307-2567-9

What the Bible Is All About
Henrietta C. Mears
Ventura, CA: Regal Books
ISBN 0-8307-24311 (Visual Edition)
      0-8307-1893-1 (*KJV*)
      0-8307-1830-3 (*NIV*)

What the Bible Says About . . .
Bob Phillips and Steve Miller
Ventura, CA: Regal Books
ISBN 0-8307-1867-2

Physical Health

ACSM Fitness Book
American College of Sports Medicine
Champaign, IL: Human Kinetics
ISBN 0-8801-1783-4

ADA Complete Food and Nutrition Guide
Roberta Larson Duyff, M.S., R.D., C.F.C.S.
American Diabetes Association
Minnetonka, MN: Chronimed Publishing
ISBN 1-5656-1098-9

Building God's Temple
Dr. Richard Couey
Edina, MN: Burgess International Group
ISBN 0-8087-4891-2

Convenience Food Facts
Arlene Monk, R.D., C.D.E.
International Diabetes Center
Minneapolis, MN: IDC Publishing
ISBN 1-8851-1536-9

Exchanges for All Occasions
Marion J. Franz, M.S., R.D., C.D.E.
International Diabetes Center
Minneapolis, MN: IDC Publishing
ISBN 1-8851-1535-0

Fast Food Facts
Arlene Monk, R.D., C.D.E.
International Diabetes Center
Minneapolis, MN: IDC Publishing
ISBN 1-8851-1542-3

Why Should I Eat Better?
Lisa Messinger
Garden City Park, NY: Avery Publishing Group
ISBN 0-8952-9508-3

Cookbooks

Brand-Name Diabetic Meals in Minutes
Alexandria, VA: American Diabetes Association
ISBN 0-9454-4876-7

Brown Bag Success
Sandra K. Nissenberg, M.S., R.D. and Barbara N.
Pearl, M.S., R.D.
Minnetonka, MN: Chronimed Publishing
ISBN 1-5656-1123-3

Down-Home Diabetic Cookbook
Greendale, WI: Reiman Publications, L.P.
ISBN 0-8982-1153-0

First Place Favorites
Nashville, TN: LifeWay Press
ISBN 0-7673-2616-4

First Place Recipes
Birmingham, AL: Oxmoor House
ISBN 0-8487-1062-2

Healthy Home Cooking
Monroeville, AL: Kitchen Towel Productions, Inc.
ISBN 0-9654-8570-6

Month of Meals #1: Classic Cooking
Alexandria, VA: American Diabetes Association
ISBN 1-5804-0014-0

Month of Meals #2: Ethnic Delights
Alexandria, VA: American Diabetes Association
ISBN 1-5804-0015-9

Month of Meals #3: Meals in Minutes
Alexandria, VA: American Diabetes Association
ISBN 1-5804-0016-7

Month of Meals #4: Old-Time Favorites
Alexandria, VA: American Diabetes Association
ISBN 1-5804-0017-5

Month of Meals #5: Vegetarian
Alexandria, VA: American Diabetes Association
ISBN 0-9454-4834-1

Snack, Munch, Nibble, Nosh Cookbook
Alexandria, VA: American Diabetes Association
ISBN 1-5804-0000-0

Vegetarian Dinner in Minutes
Linda Gassenheimer
San Francisco: Chronicle Books
ISBN 0-8118-1383-5

FREE RESOURCES

The Human Nutrition Information Service
U.S. Department of Agriculture
HNIS, 6505 Belcrest Road, Room 328-A
Hyattsville, MD 20782-2011

The National Institutes of Health
Building 1, Room 4A-21
9000 Rockville Pike
Bethesda, MD 20892

NEWSLETTERS

First Place Newsletter
7401 Katy Freeway
Houston, TX 77024
1-800-727-5223

Nutrition Action Health Letter
1875 Connecticut Ave. N.W.
Suite 300
Washington, D.C. 20009-5728

Tufts University Diet & Nutrition Newsletter
P. O. Box 57857
Boulder CO 80322-7857
1-800-274-7581

University of California, Berkeley Wellness Letter
P.O. Box 420148
Palm Coast, FL 32142

Prevention Magazine
Box 181
Emmaus, PA 18099-0181
(215) 967-5171

University of Texas Lifetime Health Letter
P.O. Box 42034-0342
1-800-829-9177

The Johns Hopkins Medical Letter
Health After 50
P.O. Box 420179
Palm Coast, FL 32142-0342

WEBSITES

http://207.211.141.25/hhf/food/
www.cspinet.org
www.firstplace.org
www.healthyhomecooking.com
www.gospellight.com
www.mayohealth.org
www.pamsmith.org
www.prevention.com
www.healthletter.tufts.edu
www.justmove.org
www.olen.com/food/
www.usda.gov/fcs/cnpp.htm
www.WellnessLetter.com

Inspiration
In Your
Mailbox
Subscribe Today!

Every newsletter gives you:
- New recipes • Helpful articles
- Food tips • Inspiring testimonies
- Coming events • And much more!

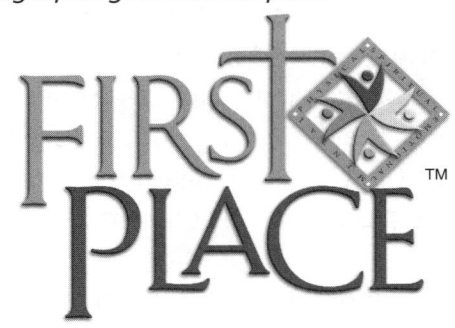

...ease enter my subscription to the First Place Newsletter.
Please print legibly. Allow 4-8 weeks for delivery of first issue.

...ne_____

...ress_____

..., State, Zip_____

...ne Phone (____)_____

...k Phone (____)_____

...il Address_____

...My check for $9.95 is enclosed; $14.99 for subscription outside continental
...A. (Please make checks payable to First Place.)

...Charge to: (circle one)

    Visa   MasterCard   Discover   American Express

...d#_____-_____-_____-_____Expires_____

...ature_____

First Place Newsletter • 7401 Katy Freeway • Houston, Texas 77024
Phone: (800) 727-5223 • Fax: (713) 688-8098 • www.firstplace.org

*Subscribe online at www.firstplace.org or
return the coupon at left.*

*Register for our free e-newsletter at
www.gospellight.com/firstplace*

FIRST PLACE ™

A Must-Have Publication for all First Place Leaders & Members!

**To receive information
about special events & products**

Stay
in the
Loop!
Register
Your Group!

First Place Group Registration Form

Your Name_____

❏ Member   ❏ Leader

Address_____

City_____State_____Zip_____

Phone Number (optional) (____) _____

E-mail Address (optional) (____) _____

Church Name _____

Church Address_____

City_____State_____Zip_____

Church Phone Number (____) _____

Church Fax Number (____) _____

Church E-mail Address _____

Name of Group Leader _____

Do you currently subcribe to the First Place newsletter? ❏ Yes ❏ No

Three Easy Ways to Register Your Group
Mail: 7401 Katy Freeway • Houston, Texas 77024
Fax: (713) 688-8098
E-mail: fpgroups@firstplace.org

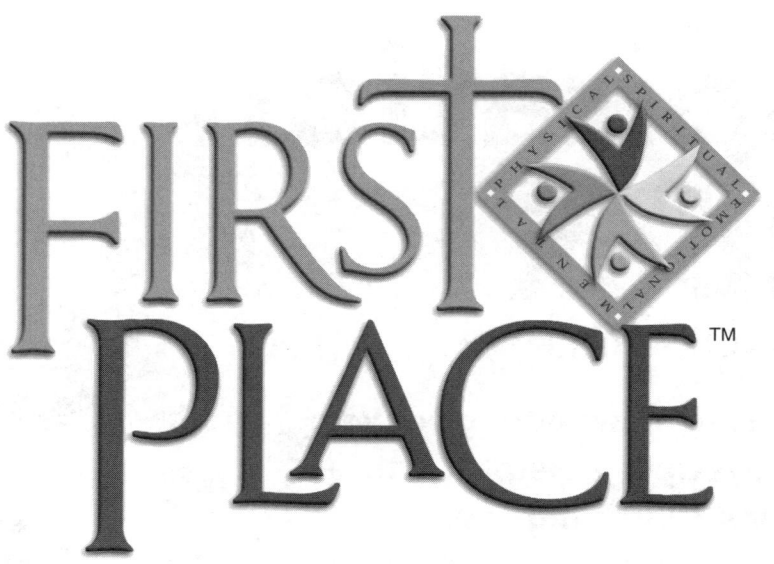

First Place was founded under the providence of God and with the conviction that there is a need for a program which will train the minds, develop the moral character and enrich the spiritual lives of all those who may come within the sphere of its influence.

First Place is dedicated to providing quality information for development of a physical, emotional and spiritual environment leading to a life that honors God in Jesus Christ. As a health-oriented program, First Place will stress the highest excellence and proficiency in instruction with a goal of developing within each participant mastery of all the basics of a lasting healthy lifestyle, so that all may achieve their highest potential in body, mind and spirit. The spiritual development of each participant shall be given high priority so that each may come to the knowledge of Jesus Christ and God's plan and purpose for each life.

First Place offers instruction, encouragement and support to help members experience a more abundant life. Please contact the First Place national office in Houston, Texas at (800) 727-5223 for information on the following resources:

- ❖ Training Opportunities
- ❖ Conferences/Rallies
- ❖ Workshops
- ❖ Fitness Weeks

Send personal testimonies to:

First Place
7401 Katy Freeway
Houston, TX 77024

Phone: **(800) 727-52223**
Website: ***www.firstplace.org***

Bible Studies
to Help You Put Christ
First

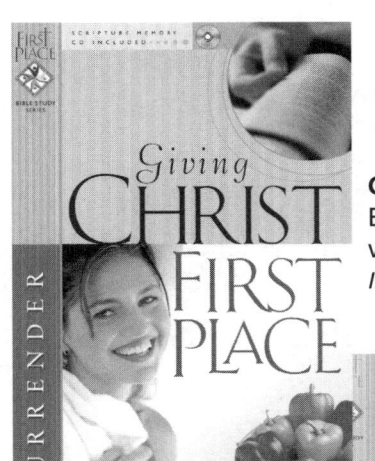

Giving Christ First Place
Bible Study
with Scripture Memory CD
ISBN 08307.28643

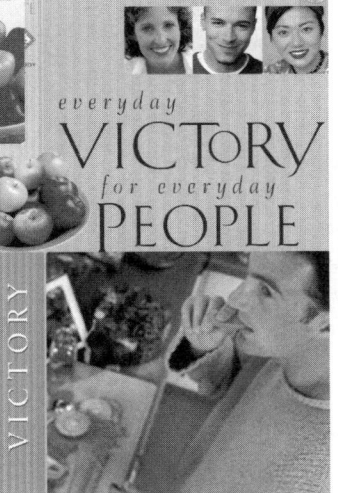

**Everyday Victory
for Everyday People**
Bible Study
with Scripture Memory CD
ISBN 08307.28651

More
Life-Changing
Bible Studies!

- **Life Under Control** - *ISBN 08307.29305 - Available January 2002*
- **Life That Wins** - *ISBN 08307.29240 - Available January 2002*
- **Seeking God's Best** - *ISBN 08307.29259 - Available April 2002*
- **Pressing On to the Prize** - *ISBN 08307.29267 - Available April 2002*
- **Pathway to Success** - *ISBN 08307.29275 - Available July 2002*
- **Living the Legacy** - *ISBN 08307.29283 - Available July 2002*

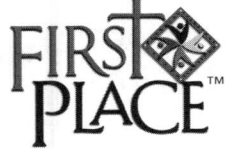

Available at your local Christian bookstore or by calling **1-800-4-GOSPEL.**

To see other First Place resources or shop online, visit **www.gospellight.com/firstplace.**

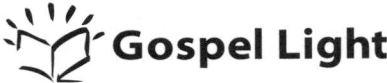